Medicine

FOR BEGINNERS

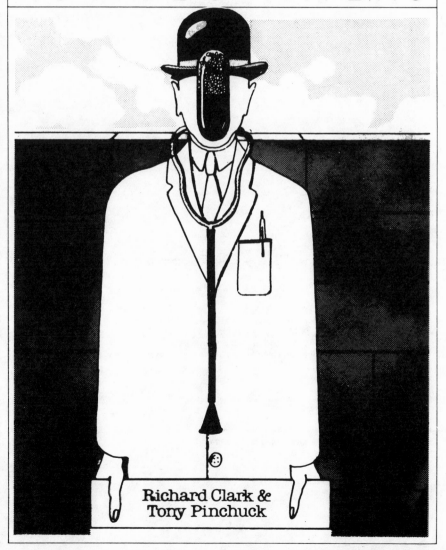

**Richard Clark &
Tony Pinchuck**

Writers and Readers

ISBN 086316 006 9
ISBN 086316 007 7 (pbk.)

A Writers and Readers Documentary Comic Book © 1984

Manufactured in the United States of America

First Edition

1234567890

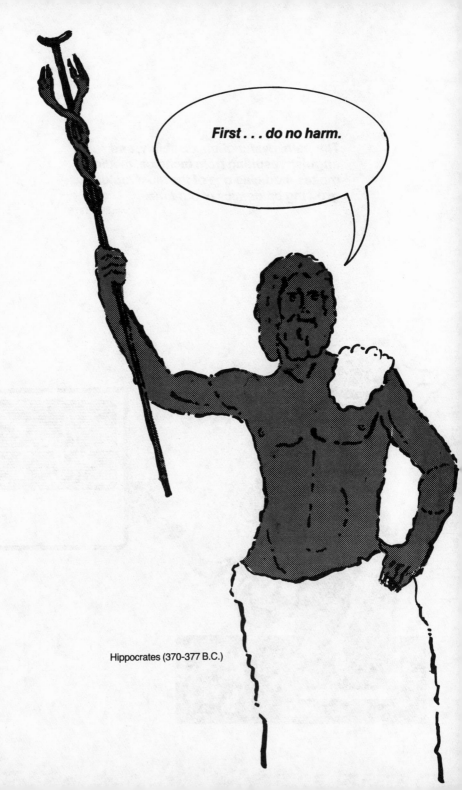

Hippocrates (370-377 B.C.)

The pain, dysfunction, disability, and anguish resulting from technical medicine makes medicine one of the most rapidly growing epidemics of our time.

Ivan Illich 1975

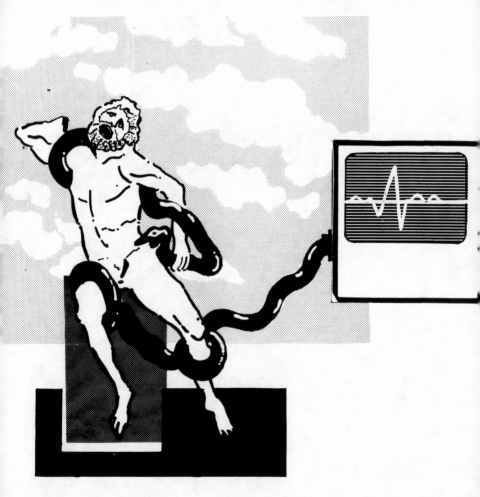

ONE

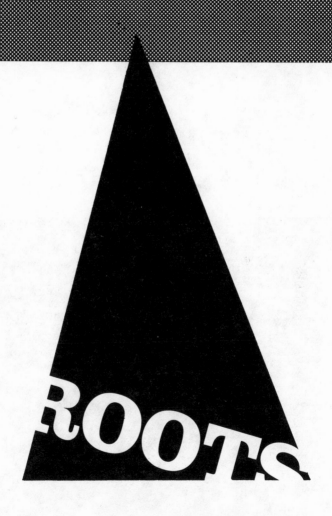

ROOTS

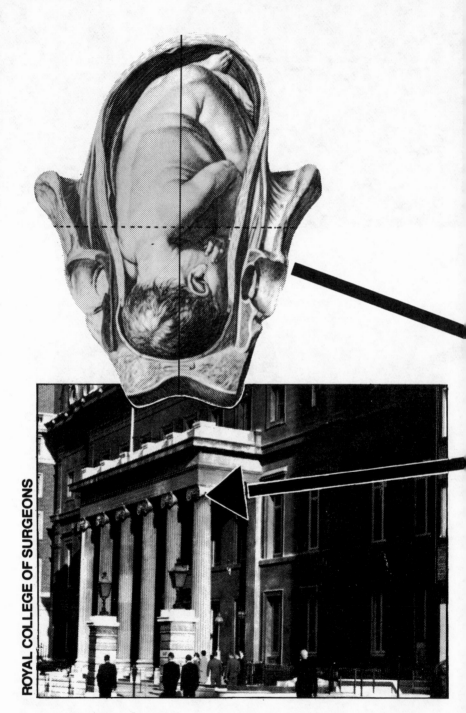

ROYAL COLLEGE OF SURGEONS

The origins of modern medicine are often traced back to the Golden Age of Greece when rationalism is said to have reigned. In those days Hippocrates lived.

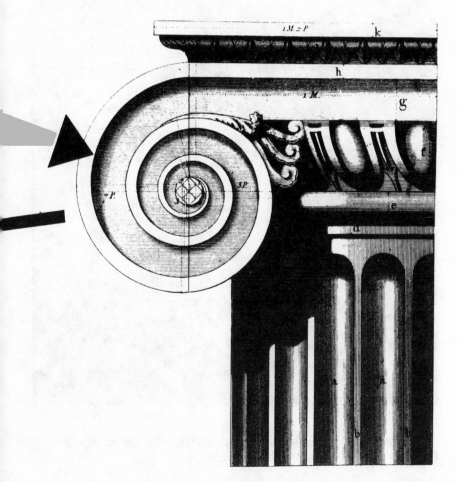

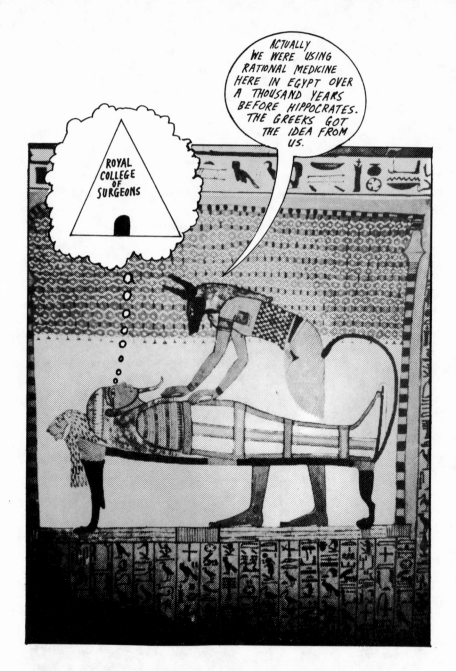

Egyptian rational medicine descended from earlier religious healing centred around the God Imhotep . . .

8

The Greeks called his counterpart Asklepios. The sick would spend a night in the god's temple where priests would treat them with bandaging, massage, or drugs. The treatments were similar to Hippocrates', which isn't surprising as the two approaches had a common origin in the Cult of Asklepios.

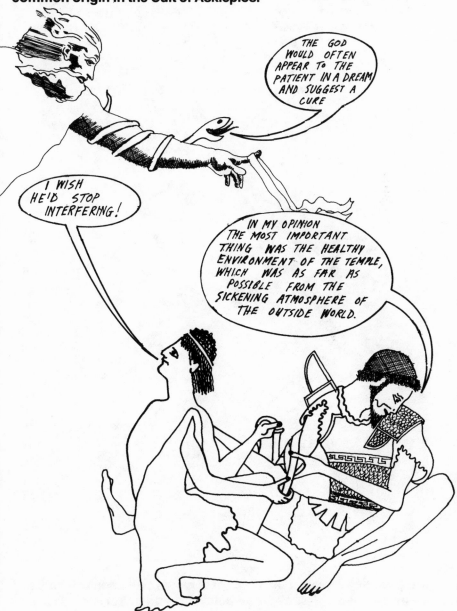

DIFFERENT APPROACHES
religious   rational

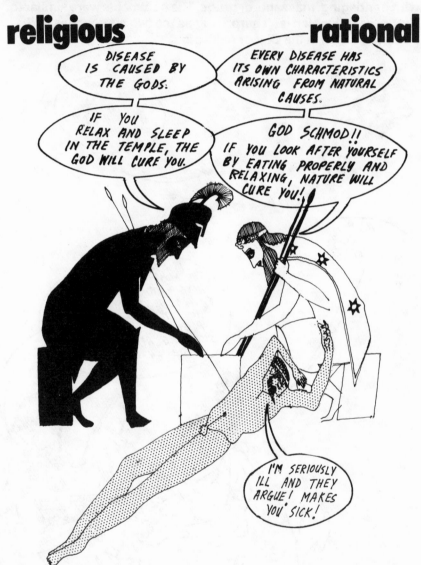

Hippocrates replaced the concept of divine causation with one of natural cause. He also made a political contribution to medicine.

The Hippocratic Oath

The first written evidence of a professional consciousness amongst medics . . .

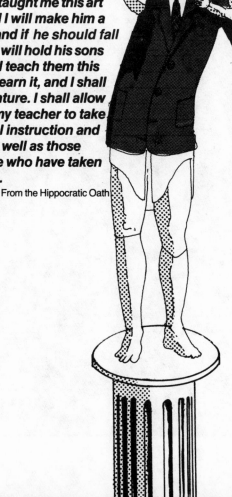

I will honour him who has taught me this art as I would my parents and I will make him a partner in my livelihood, and if he should fall into debt I will assist him. I will hold his sons as my brothers, and I shall teach them this art if they should wish to learn it, and I shall do so without fee or indenture. I shall allow my sons and the sons of my teacher to take part in my written and oral instruction and in all other instruction, as well as those pupils indentured with me who have taken the oath. But no one else.

From the Hippocratic Oath

To early Christians medical intervention was heretical. For a thousand years after Christ the approved healing was concentrated in the hands of the clergy. Meanwhile, the Arabs took up Hippocratic knowledge and developed it. In the West . . .

Hippocratic Ideas Suffered

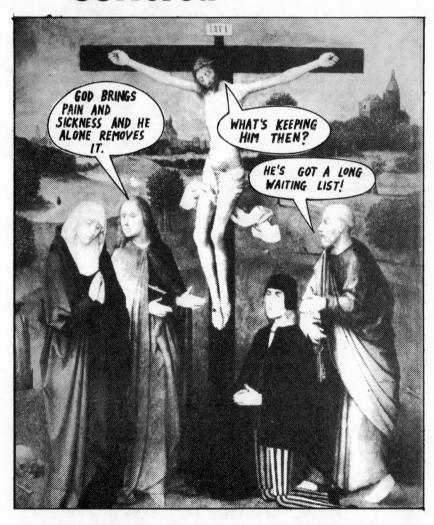

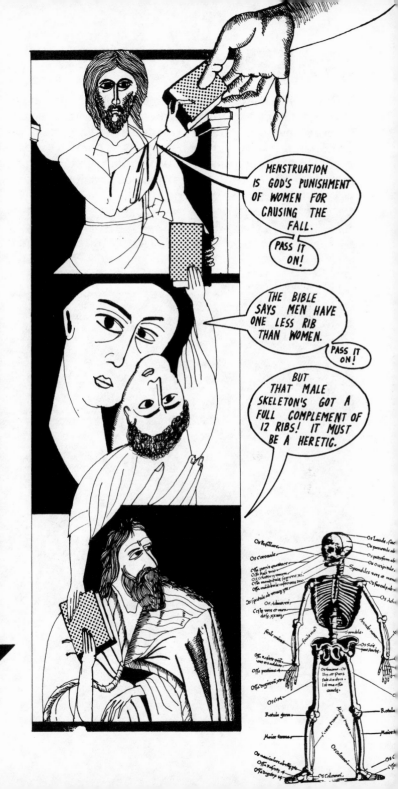

CLASSICS DUG UP

In the twelfth century an intellectual rebirth began in the West. The classical Greek and Roman writers were rediscovered, universities began to spring up and scholasticism flourished. Christian thinkers found a better way to combat the pagan heresies of the classics than prohibition. Instead of censorship, they began to incorporate as much as possible of the ancient writers into Church teachings.

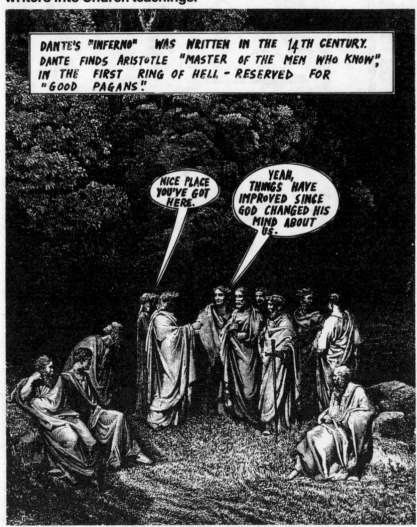

DANTE'S "INFERNO" WAS WRITTEN IN THE 14TH CENTURY. DANTE FINDS ARISTOTLE "MASTER OF THE MEN WHO KNOW" IN THE FIRST RING OF HELL - RESERVED FOR "GOOD PAGANS!"

NICE PLACE YOU'VE GOT HERE.

YEAH, THINGS HAVE IMPROVED SINCE GOD CHANGED HIS MIND ABOUT US.

CLASSICS DISCARDED

Aristotle was a follower of the school of medicine that produced Hippocrates. Aristotle's ideas became dominant in Western thought. And they posed a major obstacle to the development of modern science. Indeed the development of science and modern scientific medicine went hand in hand with the systematic overthrow of Aristotle's ideas.

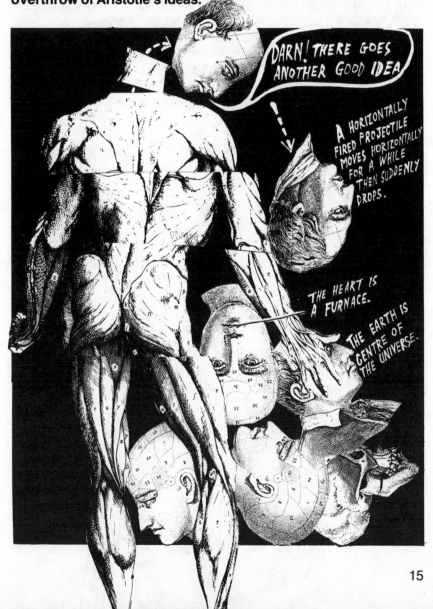

BALANCE
Life, Health, the Universe

His theory of humours was one such idea. Aristotle believed the universe was made up of the four elements: fire, air, water and earth. People were a microcosm of the universe and were composed of four humours with four corresponding personality types: blood – high spirited, yellow bile – bad tempered, black bile – melancholy, phlegm – phlegmatic. Illness was due to an imbalance of the humours. The doctor's role was to restore balance and harmonize the patient with nature;. The theory came to the West via the writings of the Roman physician, Galen. It wasn't till the middle of the 19th century that it was finally replaced by modern pathology.

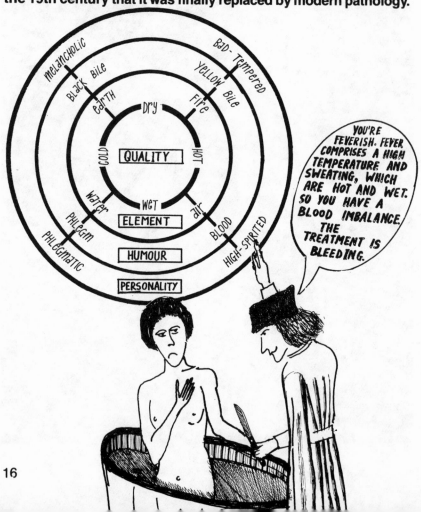

THE FALL

Aristotle's concept of *nature* was profoundly antithetical to the modern idea of science. Asked to explain why something is so, Aristotle would reply: *because that is its nature*.

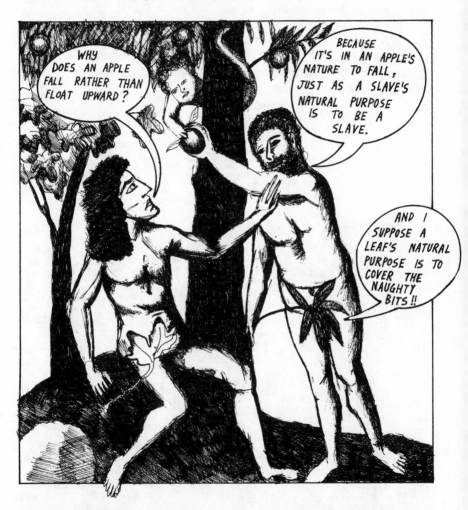

However Aristotle's philosophy had great appeal for 13th century rulers, because of its ability to justify the inequities of feudalism. Some were lords and others were serfs according to their inherent nature.

NEW VISION

The first is the eye that sees. The second the object seen. The third the distance between the two, said Albrecht Durer.

In the fifteenth century the symbolic order of the feudal world gave way to naturalistic art. By the end of the century Leonardo was producing accurate anatomical drawings. Artists became interested in perspective.

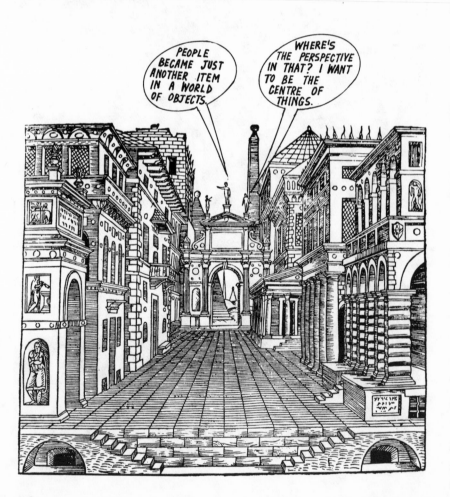

NEW ORDER

Capitalism emerged. Power shifted from the Church to secular rulers. Gunpowder, printing, and Copernicus unseated the old ways.

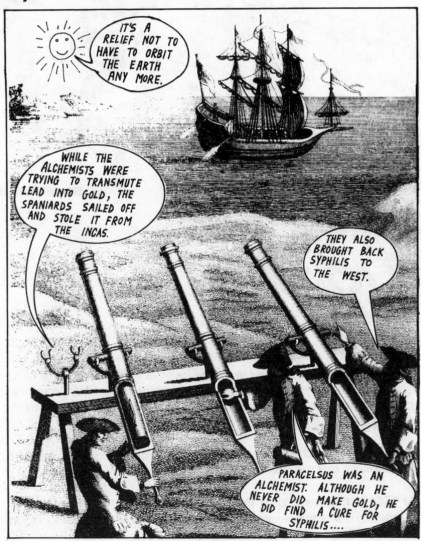

PARACELSUS

Philippus Theophrastus Bombastus von Hohenheim (1493–1541) called himself Paracelsus. Others called him bombastic. Possessed by the spirit of change, he attacked the stagnant dogmas of the medical orthodoxy and stressed empiricism.

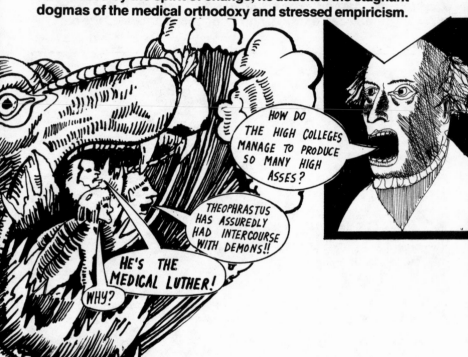

In 1517 Luther challenged the pope by nailing his Ten Theses to a church door. By pinning his lecture program to Basel University's notice board ten years later, Paracelsus opened his teaching to the public and challenged scholastic exclusiveness.

In 1520 Luther burned a papal bull excommunicating him. In 1517 Paracelsus burned the hallowed medical texts.

In 1522 Luther translated the Bible into German. Paracelsus made his lectures understandable to all by lecturing in the vernacular.

Paracelsus sowed the seeds of modern healing – both mainstream and alternative approaches.

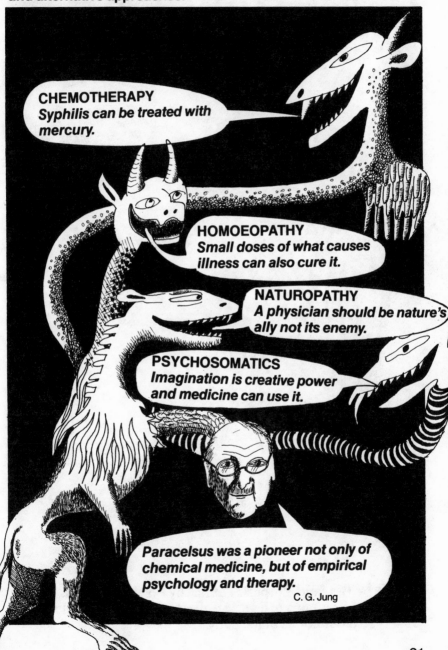

VESALIUS TURNS FROM TRADITION

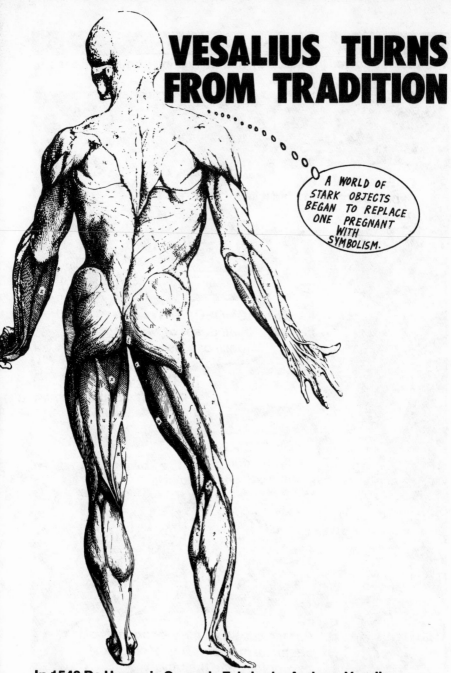

In 1543 De Humanis Corporis Fabrica by Andreas Vesalius replaced the dogmas of classical anatomy with his own closely observed illustrations of the body.

Vesalius' work heralded a renaissance in medical thinking . . .

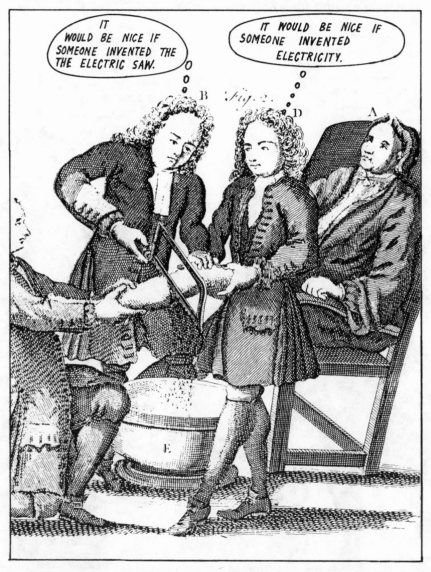

. . . which was fine in theory. But it had little impact on health till the twentieth century.

While medical technique made sluggish progress, the foundations for a scientific approach were laid. The sixteenth century saw Aristotle's world-view begin to crumble.

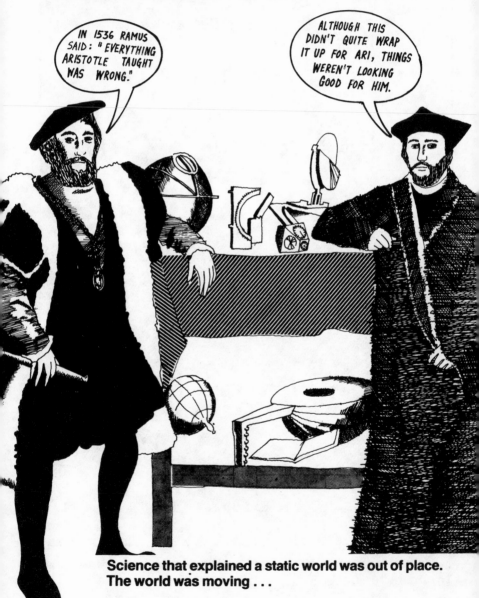

Science that explained a static world was out of place. The world was moving . . .

Experimentation

For Francis Bacon (1561–1626), Lord High Chancellor, all events were explicable in terms of matter and motion. One of the foremost proponents of the emerging science, he envisaged an ideal society run by scientists in the work: New Atlantis.

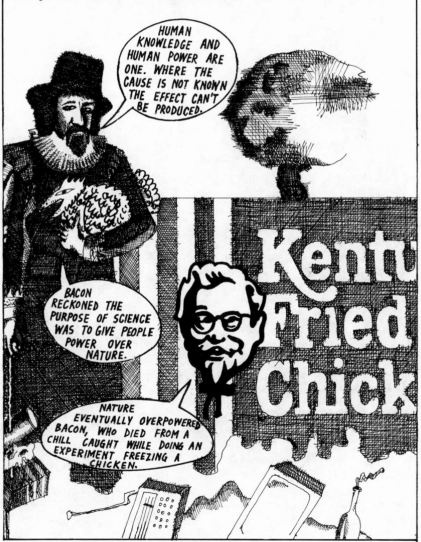

HUMAN KNOWLEDGE AND HUMAN POWER ARE ONE. WHERE THE CAUSE IS NOT KNOWN THE EFFECT CAN'T BE PRODUCED.

BACON RECKONED THE PURPOSE OF SCIENCE WAS TO GIVE PEOPLE POWER OVER NATURE.

NATURE EVENTUALLY OVERPOWERED BACON, WHO DIED FROM A CHILL CAUGHT WHILE DOING AN EXPERIMENT FREEZING A CHICKEN.

William Harvey (1578–1657) was Bacon's medical attendant. Although Harvey didn't think a lot of his employer's philosophical endeavours, he used a scientific approach to construct an hydraulic model of blood-circulation.

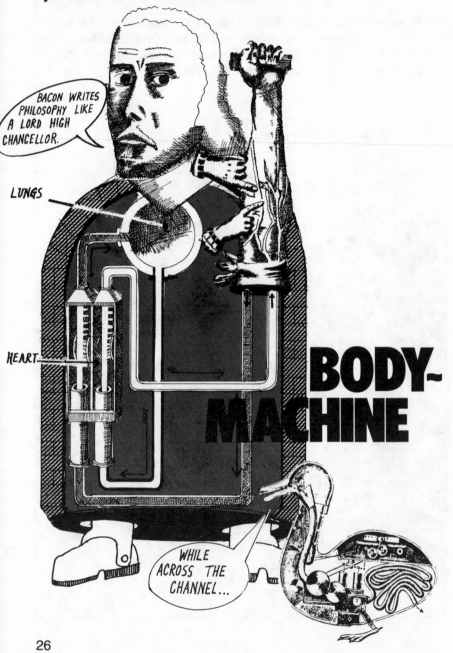

Mind Matters

René Descartes (1596–1650) applauded Harvey's discovery. Descartes and Bacon provided philosophical inspiration for the scientific revolution.

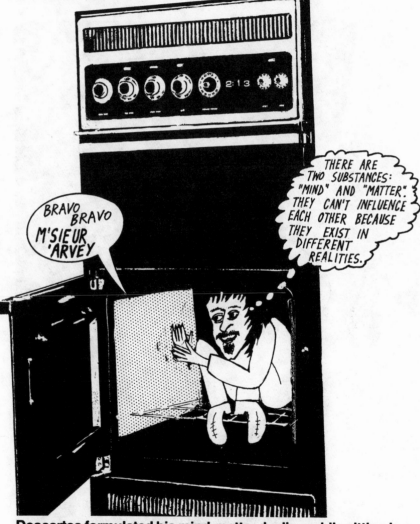

Descartes formulated his mind-matter dualism while sitting in a Dutch oven because he couldn't think when cold. His dualist theory crops up twice in modern medicine . . .

1. SCIENTIFIC METHOD

Of the two substances, mind and matter, Descartes said that only matter was suitable stuff for science to deal with. Mind's role was to stand aloof and observe matter as an object.

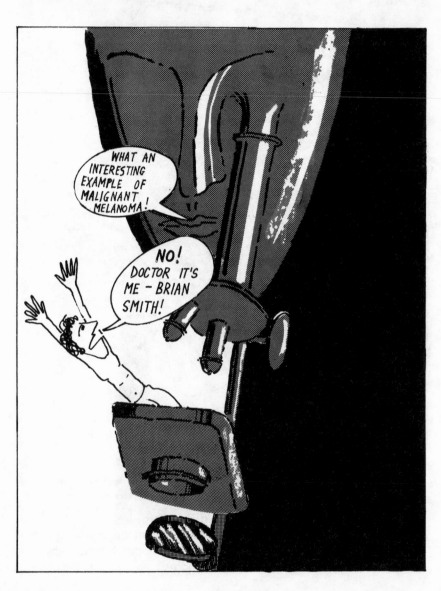

2·THE SPLIT PERSON

Animals are machines, said Descartes. Humans are machines with minds. But he also said that mind cannot interact with matter. How then, do mind and body relate?

DESCARTES' PROBLEM . . .

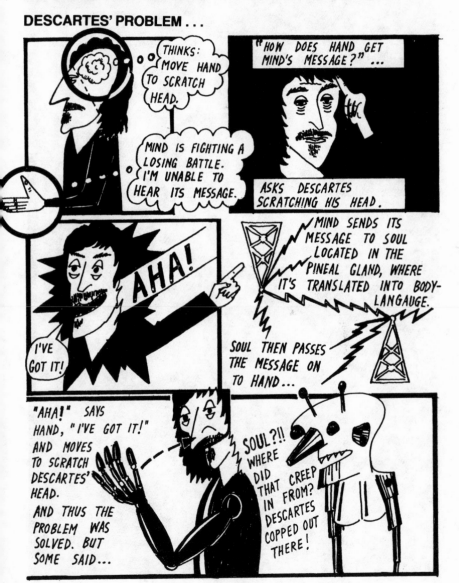

THOMAS HOBBES
arch-materialist

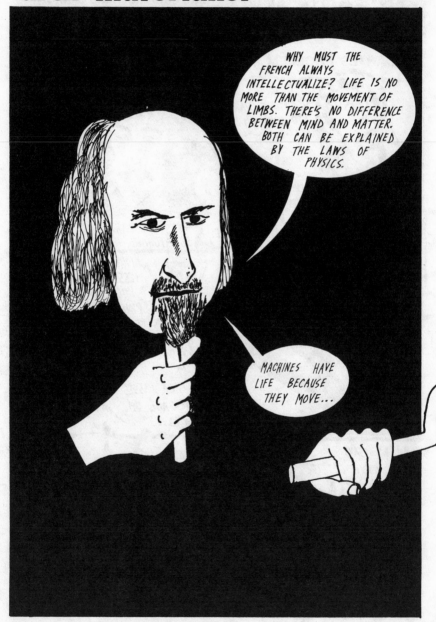

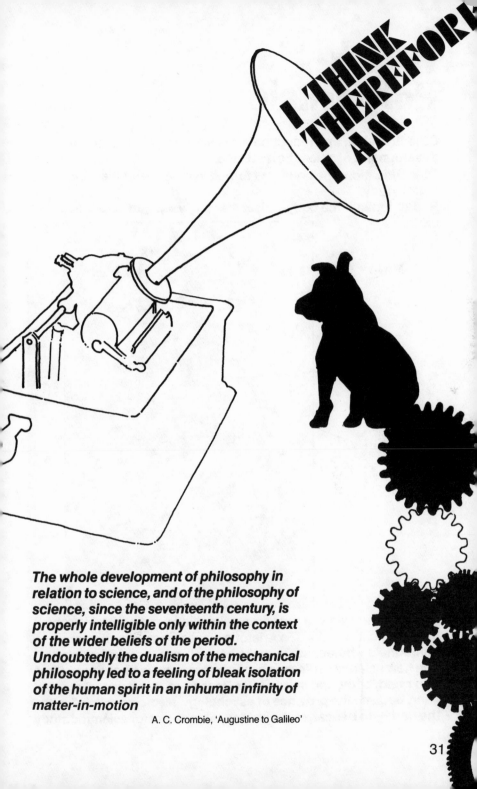

'I THINK THEREFORE I AM.'

The whole development of philosophy in relation to science, and of the philosophy of science, since the seventeenth century, is properly intelligible only within the context of the wider beliefs of the period.
Undoubtedly the dualism of the mechanical philosophy led to a feeling of bleak isolation of the human spirit in an inhuman infinity of matter-in-motion

A. C. Crombie, 'Augustine to Galileo'

31

Health·
Holy·Whole

Objectification and reductionism were prerequisites for the
development of scientific medicine.
Objectification: the body was turned into an object that science
could study.
Reductionism: the body-object was analysed into constituent
parts.

MIND

BODY

SPIRIT

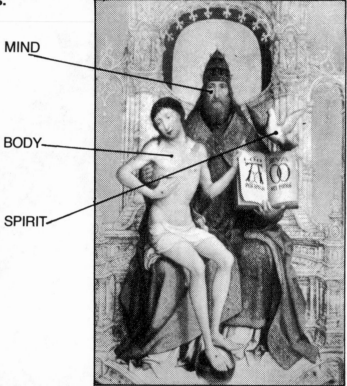

The emerging view of the person signalled a radical break from
the classical tradition. To Aristotle illness was a violation of
someone's wholeness. To make her well was to make her whole.
The new science of disease began by breaking up that whole. First
into mind, body, and spirit. After Descartes, spirit was discarded.
Mind became the province of psychology. Medicine was left with
the body – to Descartes the only suitable object for scientific study.

In the next phase medical science broke the body into smaller and smaller parts. In 1761 Giovanni Battista Morgagni (1682–1772) identified organs as the seats of disease.

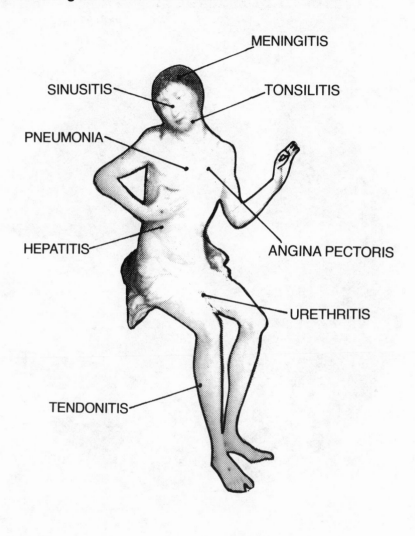

MENINGITIS

SINUSITIS

TONSILITIS

PNEUMONIA

HEPATITIS

ANGINA PECTORIS

URETHRITIS

TENDONITIS

After 1761, ill-health became less a disharmony of the individual and more like a parasitic infestation of organs by disease entities.

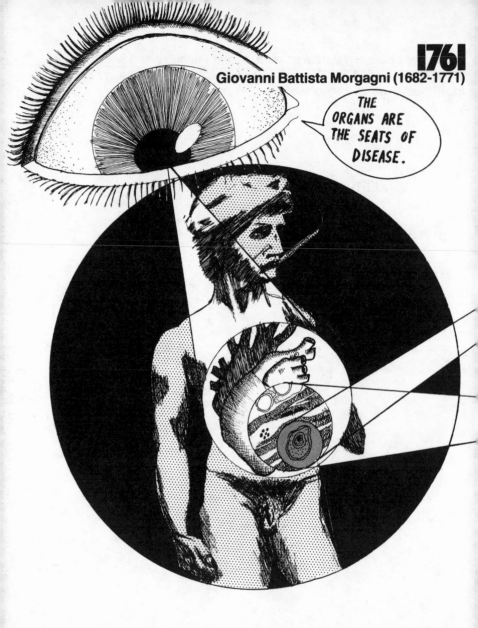

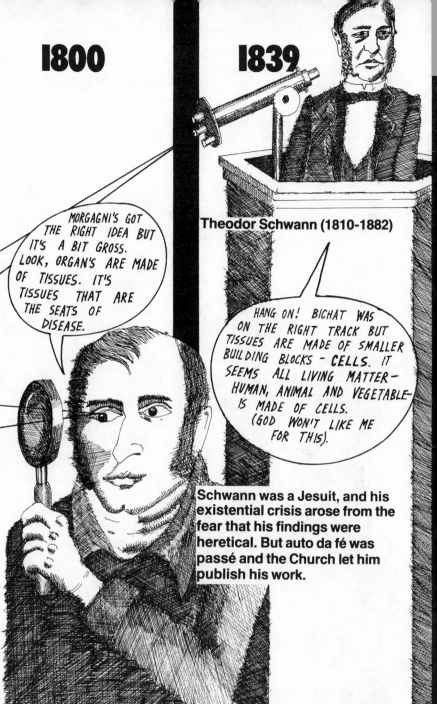

1800

1839

MORGAGNI'S GOT THE RIGHT IDEA BUT IT'S A BIT GROSS. LOOK, ORGAN'S ARE MADE OF TISSUES. IT'S TISSUES THAT ARE THE SEATS OF DISEASE.

Theodor Schwann (1810-1882)

HANG ON! BICHAT WAS ON THE RIGHT TRACK BUT TISSUES ARE MADE OF SMALLER BUILDING BLOCKS – CELLS. IT SEEMS ALL LIVING MATTER – HUMAN, ANIMAL AND VEGETABLE – IS MADE OF CELLS. (GOD WON'T LIKE ME FOR THIS).

Schwann was a Jesuit, and his existential crisis arose from the fear that his findings were heretical. But auto da fé was passé and the Church let him publish his work.

Marie François Xavier Bichat (1771-1802)

BODY POLITICS

Rudolf Virchow (1821–1902), regarded by some as the all-time greatest pathologist, struck the final death-blow to classical ideas about disease.

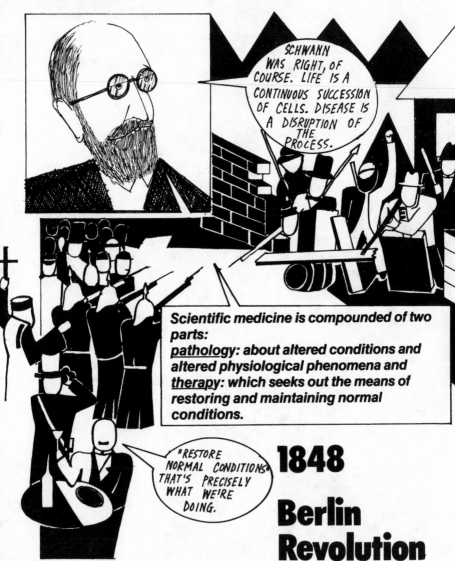

SCHWANN WAS RIGHT, OF COURSE. LIFE IS A CONTINUOUS SUCCESSION OF CELLS. DISEASE IS A DISRUPTION OF THE PROCESS.

Scientific medicine is compounded of two parts:
<u>pathology</u>: about altered conditions and altered physiological phenomena and
<u>therapy</u>: which seeks out the means of restoring and maintaining normal conditions.

"RESTORE NORMAL CONDITIONS" THAT'S PRECISELY WHAT WE'RE DOING.

1848
Berlin Revolution

Claude Bernard (1813–1878) showed that the body provides an ideal environment for cells to live in. By regulating temperature and chemical composition the body creates an interior environment which permits us to tolerate external changes while remaining internally stable. Whenever conditions change, the mechanism restores normality.

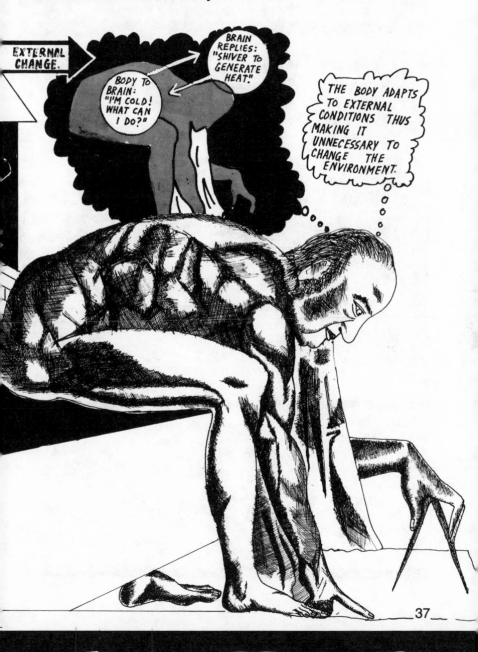

Although Virchow's cellular pathology carried medicine over the threshold of experimental science, one of the stumbling blocks, hindering practical progress was doctors' resistance to new ideas . . . as Ignaz Semmelweiss (1818–1865) discovered.

the Microbe Hunters

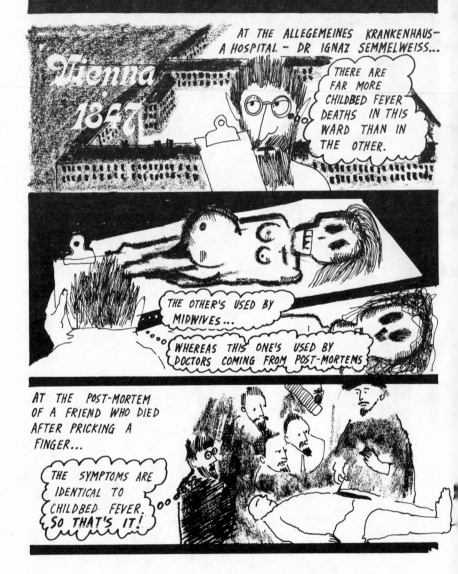

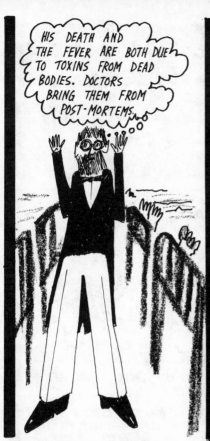

By washing his hands he reduced the mortality on his wards from 11% to 1%

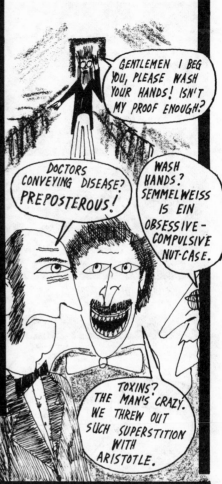

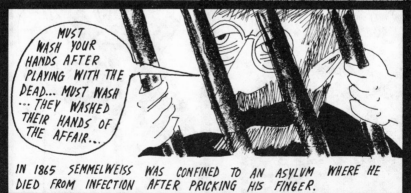

In 1865 Semmelweiss was confined to an asylum where he died from infection after pricking his finger.

the Microbe Hunters

France 1854

A DISTILLER OF ALCHOHOL APPROACHES SCIENTIST LOUIS PASTEUR.

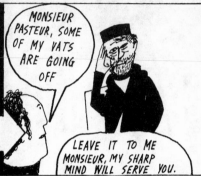

MONSIEUR PASTEUR, SOME OF MY VATS ARE GOING OFF

LEAVE IT TO ME MONSIEUR, MY SHARP MIND WILL SERVE YOU.

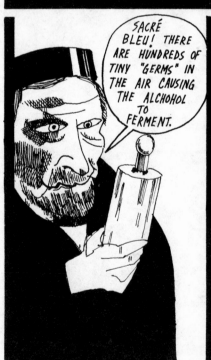

SACRÉ BLEU! THERE ARE HUNDREDS OF TINY "GERMS" IN THE AIR CAUSING THE ALCHOHOL TO FERMENT.

• IN 1861 PASTEUR PUBLISHED HIS "GERM THEORY OF DISEASE."

• IN 1870 HE IS REPUTED TO HAVE RESPONDED TO CLAUDE BERNARD'S POSTHUMOUS DENIAL OF THE GERM THEORY BY JUMPING ON THE DEAD MAN'S GRAVE.

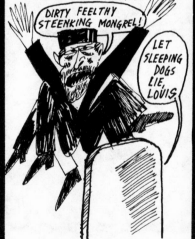

DIRTY FEELTHY STEENKING MONGREL!

LET SLEEPING DOGS LIE, LOUIS.

Glasgow 1865

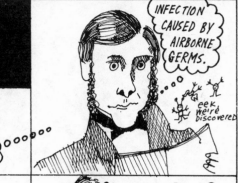

INFECTION CAUSED BY AIRBORNE GERMS.

eek we're discovered

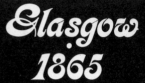

SURGEON JOSEPH LISTER READS PASTEUR'S FINDINGS.

I SAY, THIS IS INTERESTING.

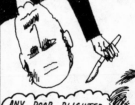

ANY POOR BLIGHTER WHO NEEDS AN OP IS MORE LIKELY THAN NOT TO DIE FROM POST-OPERATIVE INFECTION.

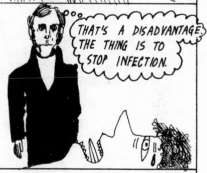

THAT'S A DISADVANTAGE. THE THING IS TO STOP INFECTION.

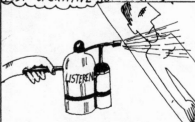

LISTERENE

LISTER ACHIEVES SUCCESS BY SPRAYING WOUNDS WITH CARBOLIC ACID.

THE IDEA TOOK DECADES TO CATCH ON IN ENGLAND.

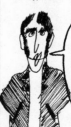

THE VERY IDEA OF SPRAYING CREOSOTE IS ANATHEMA! I'M A SURGEON AND MY PATIENTS AREN'T SPLIT-POLE FENCES!

41

The Microbes

In 1882 Robert Koch (1843–1910) identified a specific organism that causes tuberculosis. Then scientists listed others and suddenly it became apparent that the body was under siege by growing hordes.

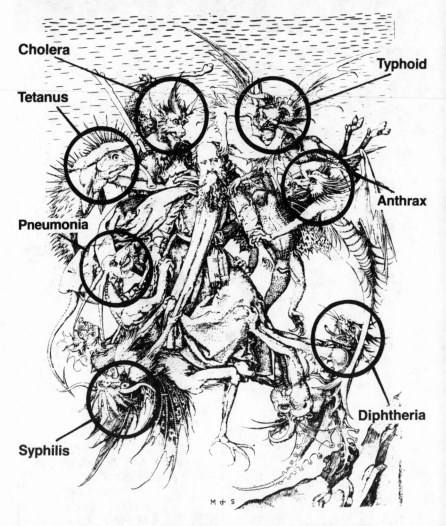

Cholera
Typhoid
Tetanus
Anthrax
Pneumonia
Diphtheria
Syphilis

Lister's response to the threat was crude. Carbolic worked because it killed all cells . . . including human tissue.

MOBILISATION!

At the turn of the century Paul Ehrlich set out in quest of the magic bullet, a chemical substance that would destroy an infective organism without harming human cells. In 1909 he found salvarsan which is effective against syphilis.

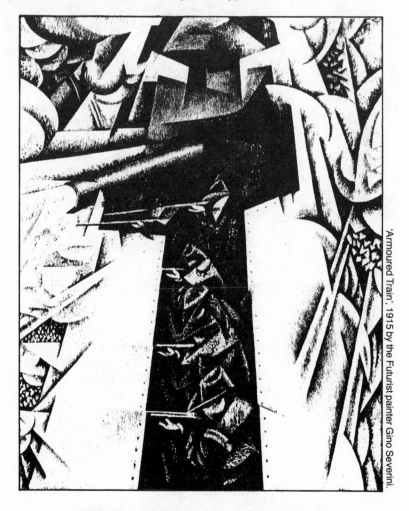

'Armoured Train', 1915 by the Futurist painter Gino Severini.

WE WILL GLORIFY WAR – THE WORLD'S ONLY HYGIENE.

From: Founding and First Manifesto of Futurism, 1909

CROSS ROAD

After the sixteenth century, medicine was broadly divided into surgery and internal medicine.

Between the sixteenth and nineteenth century neither approach showed much success in improving health. Nevertheless, by the mid-nineteenth century, medicine was well on the path to professional respectability in England and America.

SCIENCE
Surgical technique was first to benefit from the application of science. In 1844 laughing gas was used to produce analgesia. But Pasteur's germ theory was important to surgery and internal medicine.

SURGERY
1865: Lister used antiseptics – the precursor to modern surgical sterilization and aseptic techniques.

INTERNAL MEDICINE
1909: Ehrlich discovered the magic bullet, which heralded modern drugs.

Ménage à Trois

Pasteur's germ theory was a watershed for medical practice. But Pasteur himself was not a medical man and represented a third element that would mediate the doctor-patient relationship. It culminated in the dependence of doctors on scientists and equipment suppliers.

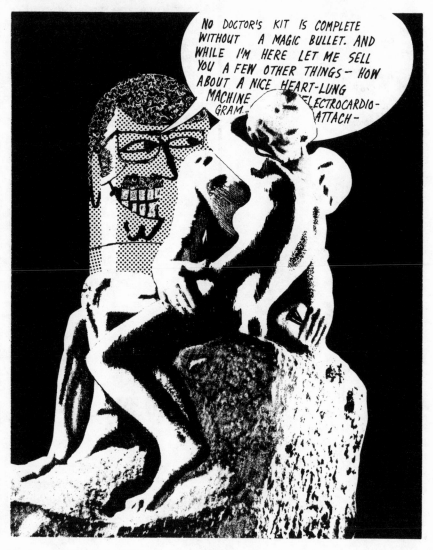

OTHER POSSIBILITIES

SAMUEL HAHNEMANN
(1755 - 1843)
ALREADY HAD A
CONSIDERABLE
REPUTATION AS A
PHARMACOLOGIST
AND DOCTOR WHEN HE
GAVE UP HIS FLOURISHING
PRACTICE.

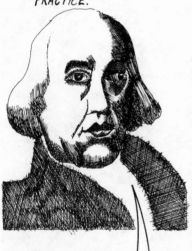

I WANTED TO STOP
INJURING MY PATIENTS.
I KNEW THERE HAD TO
BE A GENTLER AND
MORE PRECISE APPROACH
THAN THE BLUNDERBUSS
TREATMENTS USED BY
THE ALLOPATHS.

ALLOPATHY
Allopathy is the underlying principle of orthodox medical practice. In Hahnemann's time it meant balancing the four humours. For example, a patient suffering from an 'excess of blood' would be leeched by the doctor to remove some.

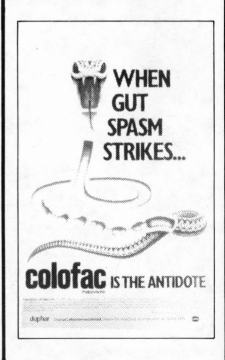

Antidotes are the basic tools of allopathy, which seeks to counteract symptoms.

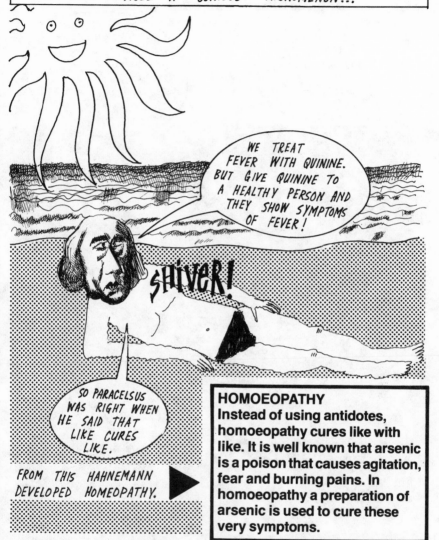

WHEN HAHNEMANN SET ABOUT BUILDING A PHARMACOPOEIA THROUGH EXPERIMENTS ON HIMSELF, HE SOON NOTICED A CURIOUS PHENOMENON...

WE TREAT FEVER WITH QUININE. BUT GIVE QUININE TO A HEALTHY PERSON AND THEY SHOW SYMPTOMS OF FEVER!

SHIVER!

SO PARACELSUS WAS RIGHT WHEN HE SAID THAT LIKE CURES LIKE.

FROM THIS HAHNEMANN DEVELOPED HOMEOPATHY.

HOMOEOPATHY
Instead of using antidotes, homoeopathy cures like with like. It is well known that arsenic is a poison that causes agitation, fear and burning pains. In homoeopathy a preparation of arsenic is used to cure these very symptoms.

For many years Hahnemann was hounded from town to town. Allopaths were not pleased with new ideas that contradicted their dogmas. Chemists didn't like the fact that homoeopathy might be bad for business.

47

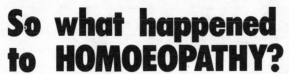

So what happened to HOMOEOPATHY?

REJECTION
without
TRIAL

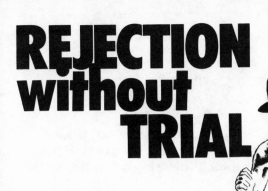

In the nineteenth century, those who could afford it went to homoeopaths. It was popular with royalty and aristocrats in Europe, and the corporate capitalists of America liked it too. But the rising medical profession did its best to suppress it. Homoeopathy became exclusive, and unavailable to most people. In England, the Queen still has a homoeopath.

Recent clinical trials indicate that homoeopathy is as effective as certain arthritis drugs, without the problem side-effects!

Homoeopathy

Science of the Times

In 1633 the Inquisition effectively ended science in Italy when it condemned Galileo for saying the earth revolves round the sun. Traditionalists refused to look through his telescope which they said revealed only delusions.

During the cholera outbreak of 1854 the Board of Health in London suppressed the fact that deaths at the homoeopathic hospital were a mere 16.4% next to the 50% average for other hospitals. When caught out, the Board explained:

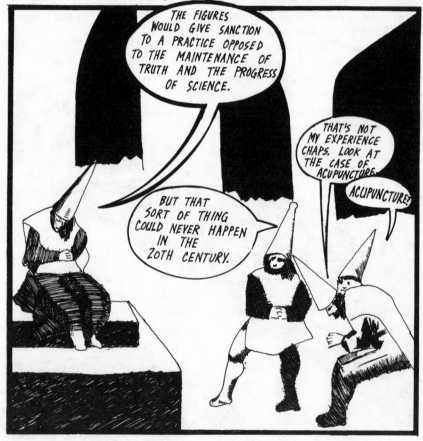

In the 1960s acupuncture was brought to Britain.

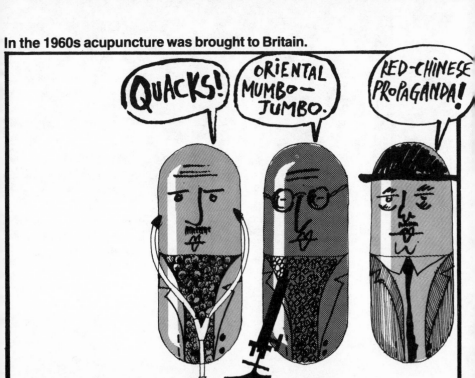

In spite of official condemnation acupuncture gained popularity. It seemed effective where orthodox treatments failed. Then it emerged that acupuncture produced anaesthesia without the usual side-effects.

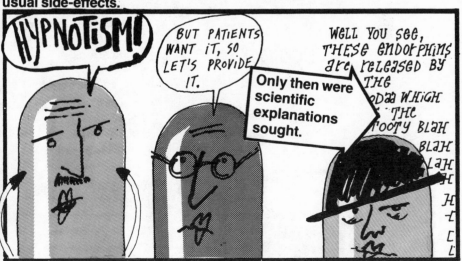

Look for the label!

scientific (adj):
1. very skilful; systematic, precise; accurate and objective.
2. based on the principles or methods of science.

scientific has replaced **christian** as the official stamp of approval.

the label **unscientific** is often used to smear an idea so it won't get a fair hearing.

Science ®
ideological application

recent tests show that the word **science** has many applications.

Science ®

Effective in promoting knowledge.

Effective in hiding it.

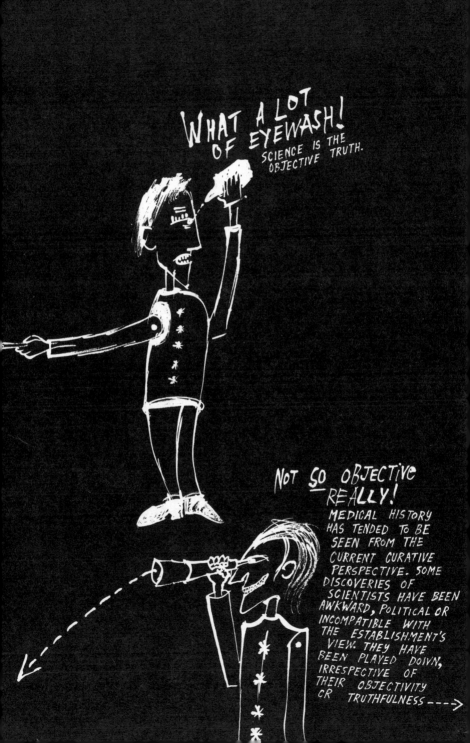

A GERM OF TRUTH

After discovering airborne infection Pasteur moved onto other things. In 1880, through curiosity he injected some chickens with cholera organisms.

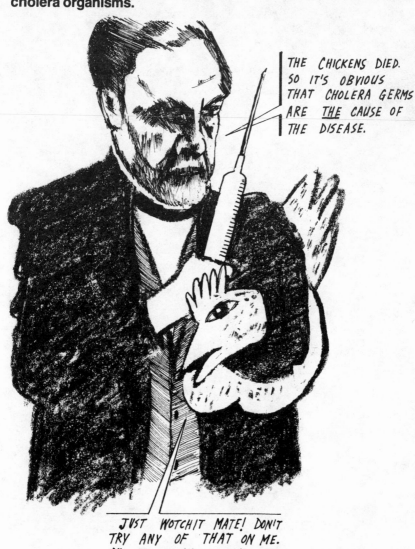

THE REAL THING

Max von Pettenkofer (1818–1901) wasn't convinced. At the ripe age of seventy-four von Pettenkofer, Professor of Hygiene at Munich University, drank a solution of pure cholera organisms for a bet, and . . . nothing happened.

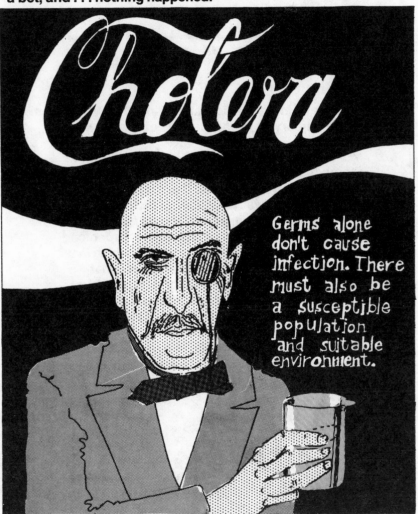

Cholera drinking became all the rage and following his trend-setting example over forty scientists imitated him.

RUDOLF VIRCHOW
POVERTY CAUSES ILLNESS

reprise... Cell Theory

Representative of many medical historians, Dr J. Miller sees Virchow's cell theory as a reflection of political views:

> *For scientists such as Virchow, the way in which cells arose and composed themselves indicated that the living organism was a republic of biological persons dividing their labours and differentiating their functions in order to serve the living commonwealth which they constituted. It is often pointed out that Virchow arrived at this conclusion under the influence of his political beliefs, and that as a passionate liberal of the 1848 generation he was predisposed to see organisms in republican terms.*

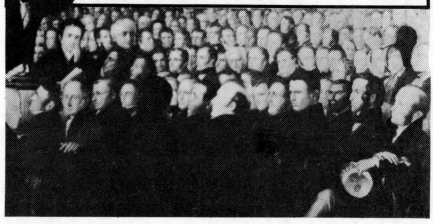

But Virchow's mixture of medicine and politics went deeper. In 1848 he was sent by the Prussian government to investigate a typhus epidemic in Silesia. He realized that the underlying causes of the outbreak were the prevailing political conditions. In his report he condemned the government and demanded social change. He was dismissed and eight days later he was at the barricades during the Berlin revolution.

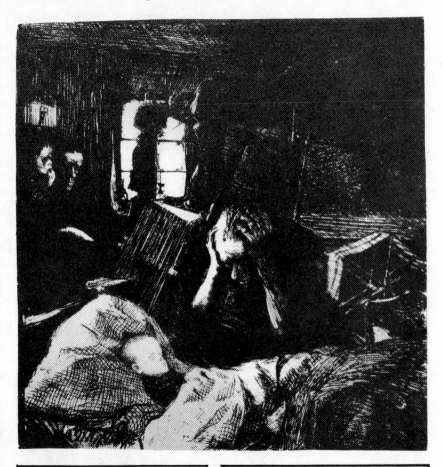

Virchow
twin action

- Scientific study of infection.
- Political causes of disease.

Nearly a hundred years later Bertolt Brecht writes:

Are you able to heal?
When we come to you
Our rags are torn off us
And you listen all over our naked body.
As to the cause of our illness
One glance at our rags would
Tell you more. It is the same cause that wears out
Our bodies and our clothes.

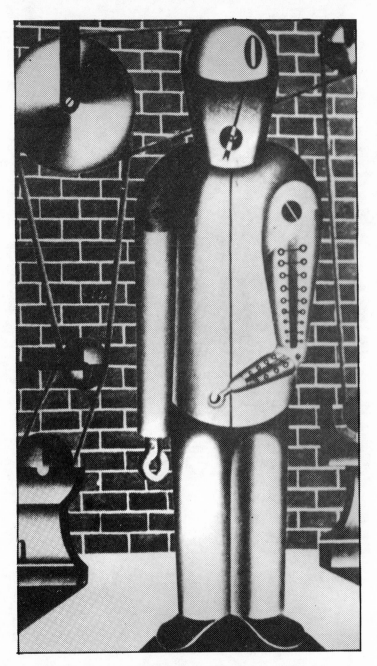

Not equipped to deal with social and political causes of disease, doctors must concentrate on individual pathology.

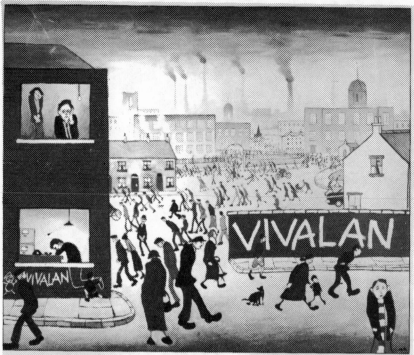

The workers' antidepressant.

When difficulty in coping with work or domestic responsibilities is a feature of depressive illness, a treatment which causes drowsiness may add to the patient's problems.

'Vivalan' is unique, improving mood and restoring drive without daytime drowsiness so that the patient is able to take a lively interest in work, social life and the family.

Listless, apathetic, tired patients who complain of fatigue and inability to concentrate are those most likely to benefit from 'Vivalan'.

  VIVALAN
The workers' antidepressant.

60

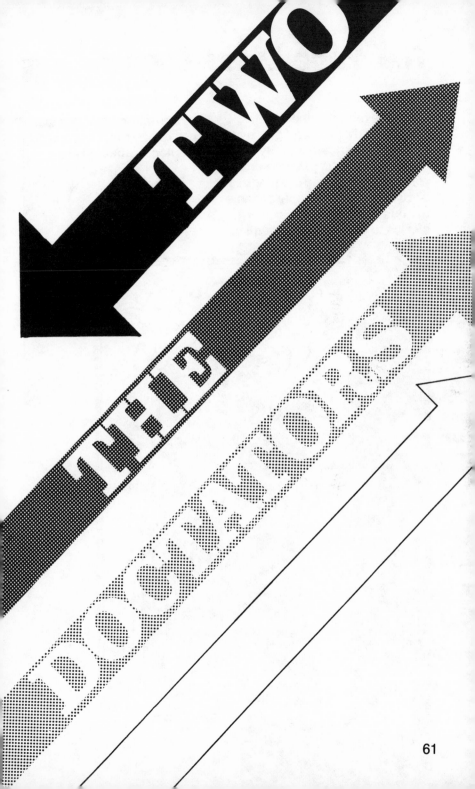

TWO
THE
DOCTATORS

The Pope Loses Control

Up to the renaissance the Church had a powerful grip over healing and knowledge. By the fourteenth century its power was waning. During the plagues of 1348 and 1381 people became disillusioned by the failure of clerics to control the epidemics.

The reputation of clerics wasn't improved by their mass exodus from plague affected areas.

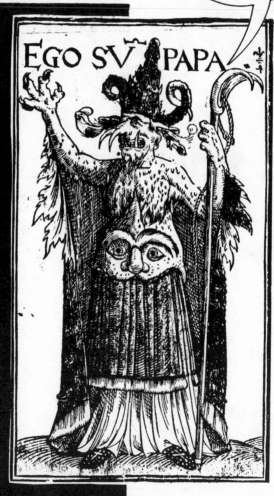

Henry VIII Steps In

In England the crown filled the vacuum left by the church. Lay-healers and the new political order needed to rework their relationship.

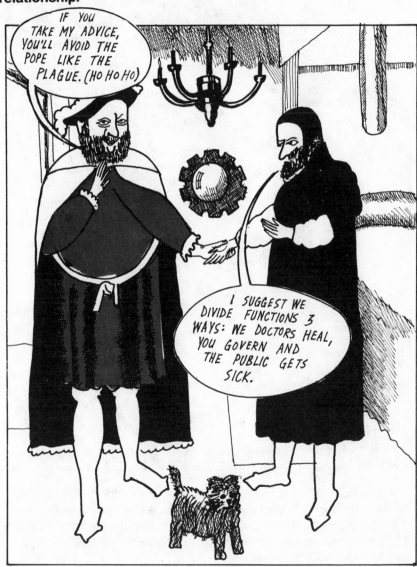

MONOPOLY
GETS A BOOSTER

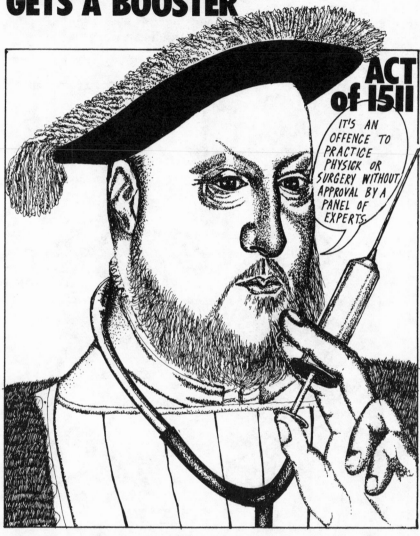

The medical elite gained further official recognition when Henry ratified the formation of the Royal College of Physicians in 1518. The College was given power to fine unauthorized practitioners. In 1540 barbers and surgeons got similar powers when the king approved their Company.

QUACKS DUCK

Without delay the barber-surgeons used their powers to persecute unauthorised practitioners. These 'quacks' were healers who relied on traditional knowledge of herbs and healing. Most were poor and served the poor. And it was the poor who suffered through their suppression.

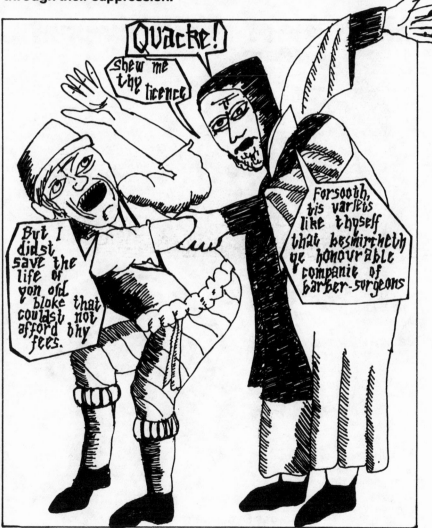

MALPRACTICE

So ruthless was the persecution that within two years there were insufficient healers. So in 1542 Henry enacted the Quack's Charter which exempted many unauthorized practitioners from the 1511 Act.

Many great minds thought...

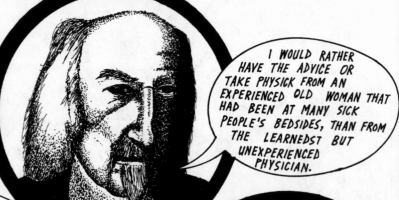

I WOULD RATHER HAVE THE ADVICE OR TAKE PHYSICK FROM AN EXPERIENCED OLD WOMAN THAT HAD BEEN AT MANY SICK PEOPLE'S BEDSIDES, THAN FROM THE LEARNEDST BUT UNEXPERIENCED PHYSICIAN.

Thomas Hobbes

ACADEMIC MEDICINE IS MERE CONJECTURE AND IS THEREFORE USELESS.
James I

EMPIRICS AND OLD WOMEN ARE MORE HAPPY MANY TIMES IN THEIR CURES THAN LEARNED PHYSICIANS

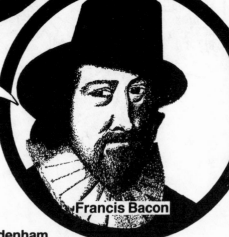

Francis Bacon

THE ART OF PHYSICK IS HAZARDOUS. MANY POOR MEN OWE THEIR LIVES TO THEIR INABILITY TO AFFORD PHYSICIANS FEES.

**Thomas Sydenham
(leading 17th century physician)**

66

WITCHES
DOCTORED

No sooner had he taken the screws off the 'quacks' than the king passed the First Penal Law against witches. The medical elite shifted their target from the poor in general, to women in particular. In 1584 Reginald Scot commented:

> *At this day it is indifferent to say she is a witch or she is a wise woman.*

Witches provided a convenient scapegoat for the medical establishment.

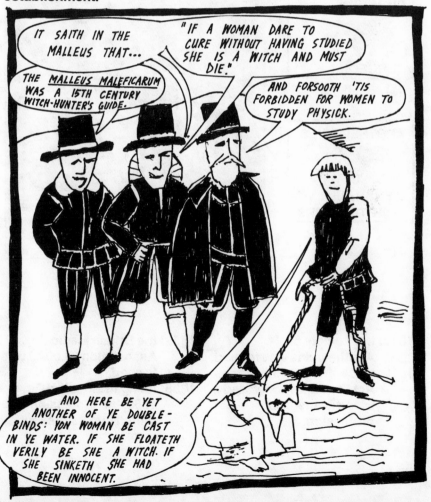

TRINITY

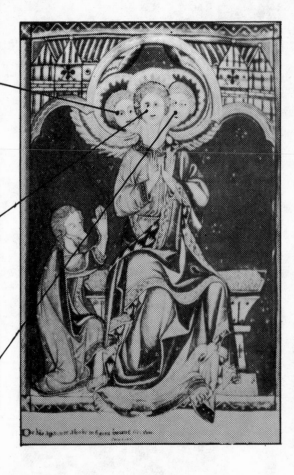

PHYSICIANS
PHYSICIANS

BARBER—SURGEONS
SURGEONS

APOTHECARIES
▼
GENERAL PRACTITIONERS

1617: the Society of Apothecaries was formed.

1815: through the Apothecaries Act the state recognized a tripartite medical profession.

1832: the British Medical Association (B.M.A.) was formed.

1858: using the Medical Act of 1858, the profession united into its present form.

Deaths on decline
1832: BMA formed

Between 1800 and 1980 the population of England grew from nine million to over fifty million. This went hand in hand with the decline of a small group of infectious diseases. The medical profession galloped in to take the credit.

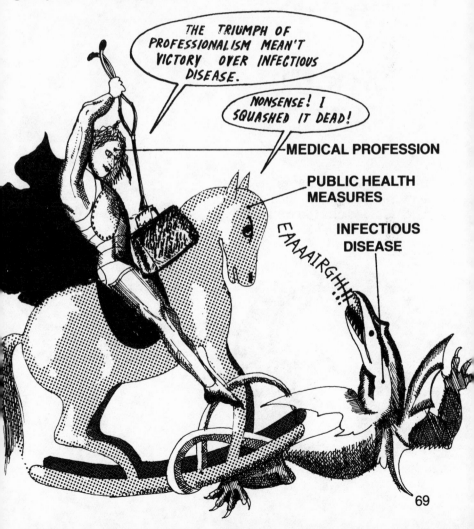

THE TRIUMPH OF PROFESSIONALISM MEAN'T VICTORY OVER INFECTIOUS DISEASE.

NONSENSE! I SQUASHED IT DEAD!

MEDICAL PROFESSION

PUBLIC HEALTH MEASURES

INFECTIOUS DISEASE

EAAAAIRGHH...!!!

WOMEN get THE TREATMENT

!

After 1858 any authorised doctor had to be on the medical register. The first edition of the register in 1859, contained the name of just one woman – Elizabeth Blackwell.

WOMEN! KEEP 'EM OUT! BATTEN THE HATCHES CHAPS.

In 1859 Elizabeth Garrett heard a lecture by Elizabeth Blackwell and decided she too would qualify in medicine.

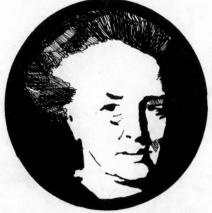

But no medical school would admit her for tuition and nobody would let her take the exams.

So Garrett took private instruction and, using a legal loophole, got herself admitted to the apothecaries exam.

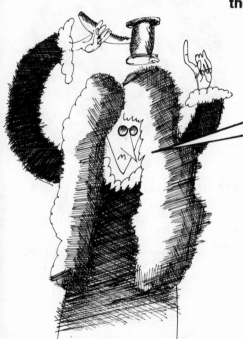

THE ACT SAYS: "ALL PERSONS WHO HAVE FULFILLED APPRENTICESHIP MUST BE ADMITTED TO THE EXAMINATION."

She passed the exam in 1865 and was entered in the medical register. The law was quickly changed to stop other women doing the same.

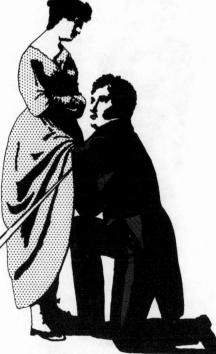

MEDICINE'S NO CAREER FOR A GIRL.

THE VERY THOUGHT IS IMPROPER.

But in 1869 a third woman took on the profession. Sophia Jex-Blake was rejected by London University. After repeatedly applying, she was admitted with four others to Edinburgh University. The women studied under harassment for three years.

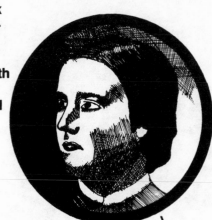

THEN in 1873

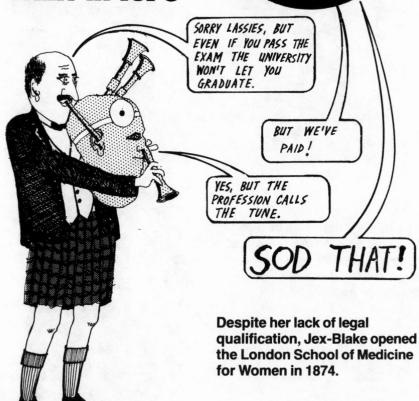

Despite her lack of legal qualification, Jex-Blake opened the London School of Medicine for Women in 1874.

SO in 1876

AN INDEPENDENT WOMEN'S MEDICAL SCHOOL? GOOD GOD - NO! UNBATTEN THE HATCHES CHAPS. GET 'EM INSIDE.

The Medical Act of 1876 opened the medical profession to women.

YET in 1976

only twenty per cent of doctors were women.

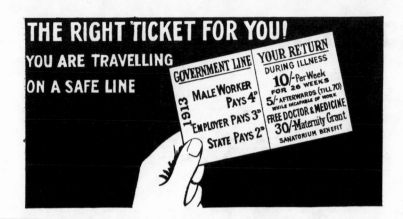

THE RIGHT TICKET FOR YOU!
YOU ARE TRAVELLING
ON A SAFE LINE

GOVERNMENT LINE
1913
MALE WORKER PAYS 4ᴅ
EMPLOYER PAYS 3ᴅ
STATE PAYS 2ᴅ

YOUR RETURN
DURING ILLNESS
10/- Per Week
FOR 26 WEEKS
5/- AFTERWARDS (TILL 70)
WHILE INCAPABLE OF WORK
FREE DOCTOR & MEDICINE
30/- Maternity Grant
SANATORIUM BENEFIT

NATIONAL HEALTH INSURANCE ACT 1911

One aim of the Act was to ensure medical care for workers.

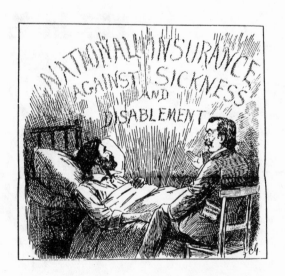

The liberal spirit?

In fact Britain wasn't first to provide health insurance. Back in 1883, Bismarck (not your average mister nice guy) set up the Sickness Insurance Act in Germany.

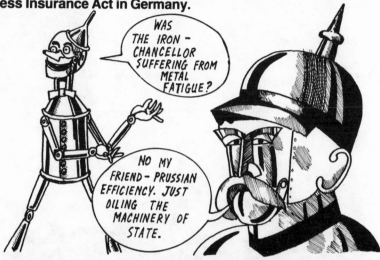

Like Lloyd George, Bismarck was reacting to social pressure.

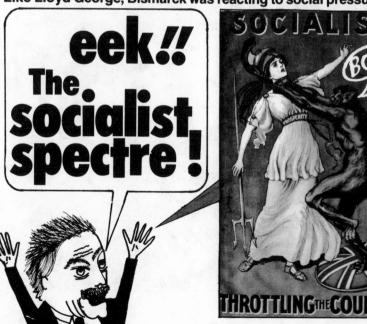

A TOUCH OF CLASS

In the 1890s trade union membership increased. Militancy and strikes became more frequent. The government was haunted by the spectre of socialism. Different leaders hit out as they thought best.

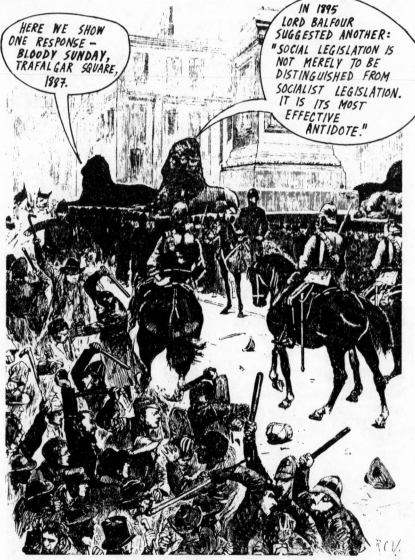

ILL WORKERS WORK ILL

Capitalism entered a new phase. New machines needed more skilled operators. Healthier workers were more productive and therefore more profitable.

The Boer War brought home the poor health of British workers. Recruitment standards were repeatedly lowered between 1883 and 1902. But large numbers of recruits were still rejected because of their feeble physique. It took three years and £250 million to defeat a bunch of farmers. What was bad for war was bad for industry.

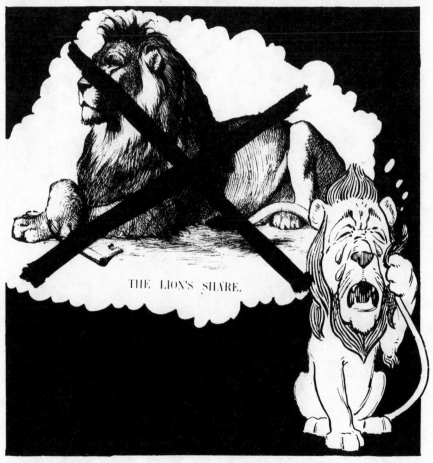

THE LION'S SHARE.

A scheme to promote the health of workers looked like a good investment.

BMA resists...

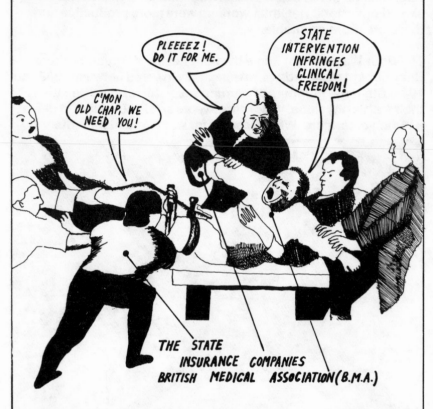

then desists

They did demand it, and the government gave in. And clinical freedom was assured, so the scheme went ahead.

What about the workers?

1911... James Keir Hardie, Labour campaigner, speaks out...

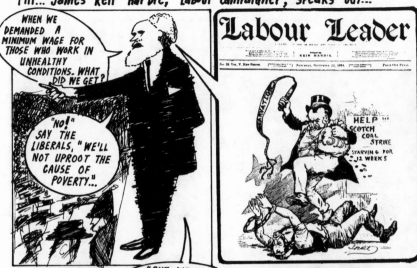

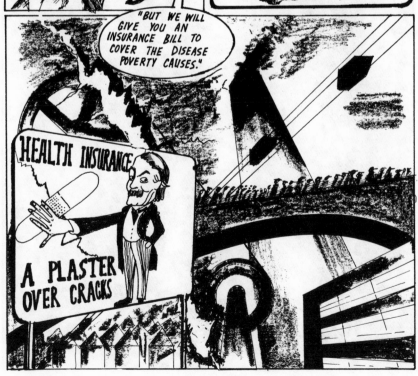

1930s DEPRIVATION

The social security offered by the National Health Insurance Act only covered those in work. With unemployment high, it failed to be an effective safety-net.

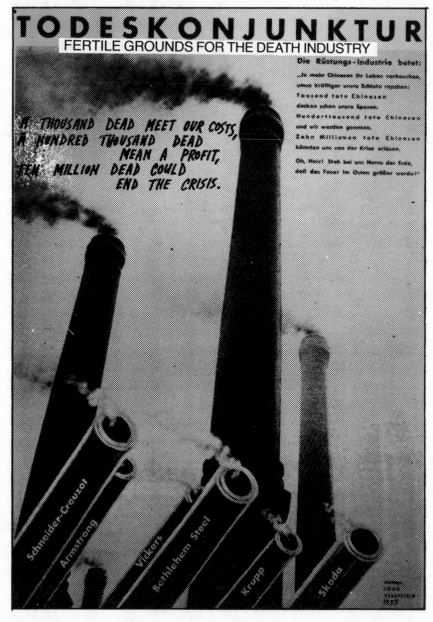

1934 LABOUR MANIFESTO

- A national health service.
- Preventive and curative.
- Open to everyone.
- Efficient and up-to-date.
- Full-time, salaried doctors.

THE BMA REACTED... SO DID TORIES:

1938 BMA recommends

- National health insurance to be extended to all workers.
- Hospitals to co-operate, not to be incorporated into a national service.
- No salaried service.

1942 Report

Churchill wasn't quite sure that workers really believed the Second World War was their battle. He thought it a good idea to convince them that post-war Britain would be better for them, that this time things would be different. In 1942 Lord Beveridge presented to Churchill a report recommending the creation of a welfare state. One of the suggestions was for a free health service for all.

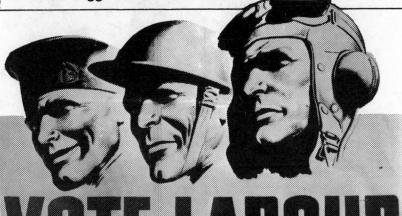

VOTE LABOUR

After the war...

Labour was swept into power with a mandate for radical reform. In 1946 the new government published the National Health Services Bill. Minister of Health, Aneurin Bevan formed an alliance with hospital consultants – the elite of the profession.

HOSPITAL CONSULTANTS

I won over the consultants by choking their mouths with gold.

Nye Bevan

A CONVERSATION BETWEEN BEVAN AND LORD MORAN (THEN-PRESIDENT OF THE ROYAL COLLEGE OF PHYSICIANS)...

BEVAN

HOW D'YOU GET A MAN TO LEAVE HIS TEACHING HOSPITAL AND GO INTO THE PERIPHERY?

MORAN

OH THEY'LL GO IF THEY GET AN INTERESTING JOB AND THEIR FINANCIAL FUTURE IS SECURED BY A PROPER SALARY.

ONLY THE STATE COULD PAY THOSE SALARIES. THIS WOULD MEAN THE NATIONALIZATION OF HOSPITALS.

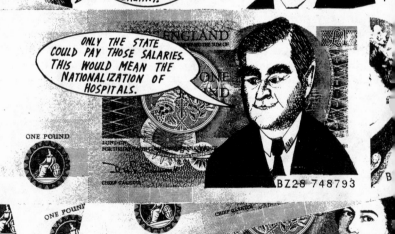

GENERAL PRACTITIONERS

Bevan met opposition from the British Medical Association, which mainly represented G.P. interests. As in 1911, the Association was concerned about clinical freedom. It also demanded financial security for its members without the restrictions of salaried employment by the state.

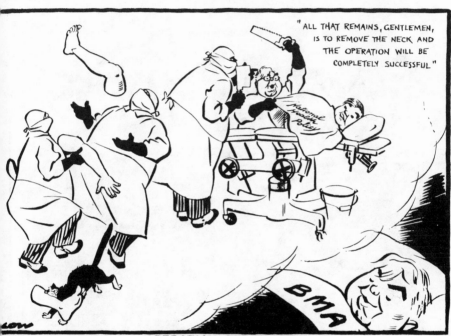

OPERATION SABOTAGE

PATIENTS

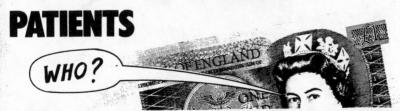

The health service Labour conceived in 1934 was far-reaching in scope. The one it delivered in 1948 looked different. It was progressive in extending a more comprehensive health insurance to everyone. But it was hardly radical.

The consultants, more than anyone, gained from Bevan's Act. It reinforced the existing medical class system. Consultant salaries grew and power became centred in their hospitals. By 1974 over two-thirds of the N.H.S. budget went to hospitals.

> *It's a marvellous health service for those that are excitingly ill, not desperately ill —* *you mustn't die boringly for the consultants.*

R.H.S. Crossman,
Secretary of State for Social Services: 1969-1970

General Practice
condition: chronic

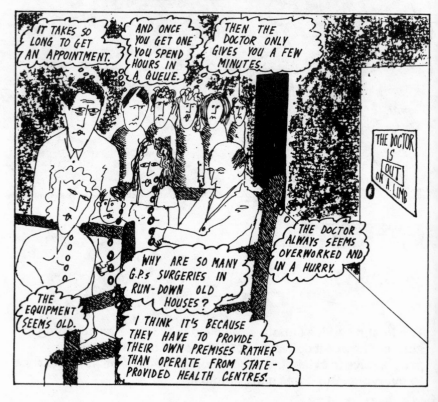

Socialism jettisoned

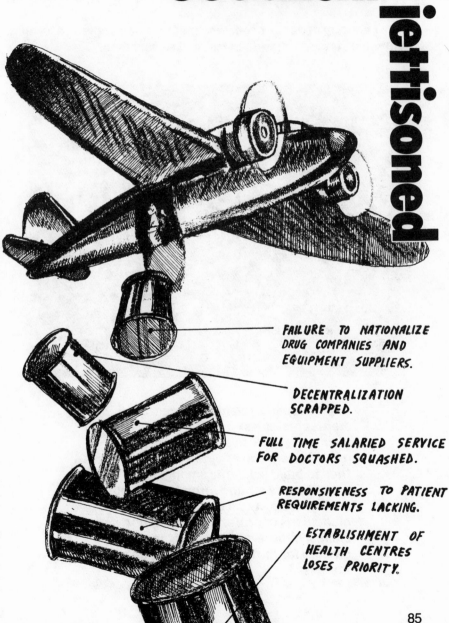

FAILURE TO NATIONALIZE
DRUG COMPANIES AND
EQUIPMENT SUPPLIERS.

DECENTRALIZATION
SCRAPPED.

FULL TIME SALARIED SERVICE
FOR DOCTORS SQUASHED.

RESPONSIVENESS TO PATIENT
REQUIREMENTS LACKING.

ESTABLISHMENT OF
HEALTH CENTRES
LOSES PRIORITY.

In 1847 a group of doctors followed the British example and formed themselves into the American Medical Association.

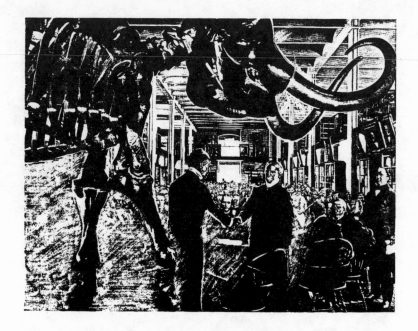

Any occupation wanting professional status creates a systematic body of theory. It claims the exclusive authority of its practitioners and adopts a code of ethics. It tries to build solidarity amongst its practitioners around formal values, norms and symbols. And it cloaks itself with the medallions of professions to support its claims. If there is no body of theory, it is created for the purpose of being able to say there is.

Eliot Freidson quoted in 'Rockefeller Medicine Men'

Nineteenth century America had several competing medical approaches. No single school of thought was dominant. It was so easy to become a doctor that there was a glut on the market, leaving most poor.

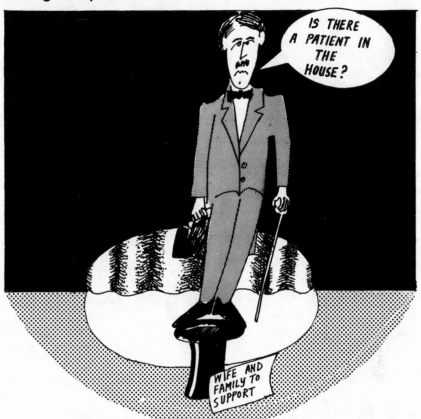

Who's «TOP DOC»?

The nineteenth and early twentieth century saw the regulars fight for monopoly. The regulars were allopaths, who treated the middle classes. Their middle-class constituency gave them an advantage over the rest . . .

At the turn of the last century, the regulars used their influence to have laws passed in state legislatures.

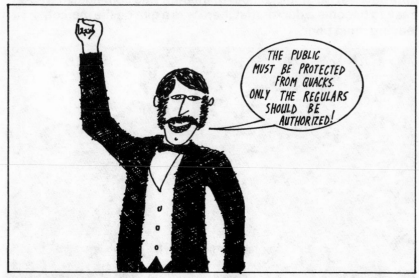

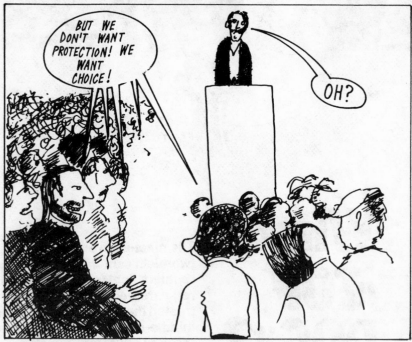

By the middle of the century the laws had been repealed.

The reversal was forced by a rising tide of populism.

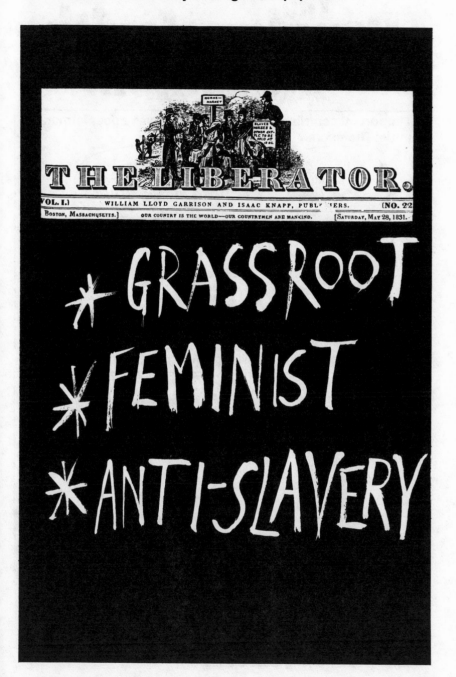

The Popular Health Movement

An important contributor to the movement was a poor farmer, Samuel Thomson.

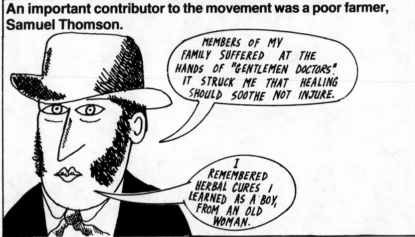

MEMBERS OF MY FAMILY SUFFERED AT THE HANDS OF "GENTLEMEN DOCTORS". IT STRUCK ME THAT HEALING SHOULD SOOTHE NOT INJURE.

I REMEMBERED HERBAL CURES I LEARNED AS A BOY, FROM AN OLD WOMAN.

In 1822 he recorded the knowledge in a book.

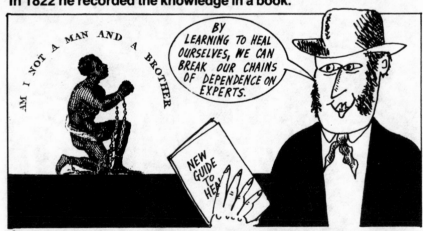

BY LEARNING TO HEAL OURSELVES, WE CAN BREAK OUR CHAINS OF DEPENDENCE ON EXPERTS.

AM I NOT A MAN AND A BROTHER

NEW GUIDE TO HEAL

By 1839, a hundred thousand copies of his New Guide to Health had been sold. At its peak, Thomsonianism embraced nearly a quarter of Americans. It was democratic in giving people power and knowledge to heal themselves. It was political in pushing women's and working class issues.

90

But in 1838 Alva Curtis split from the annual Thomsonian convention and established the Independent Thomsonian Botanical Society . . .

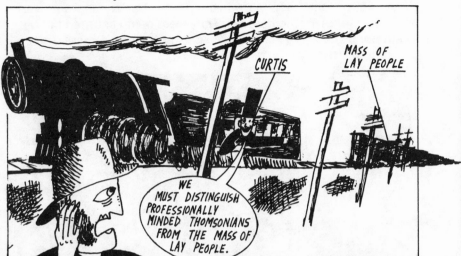

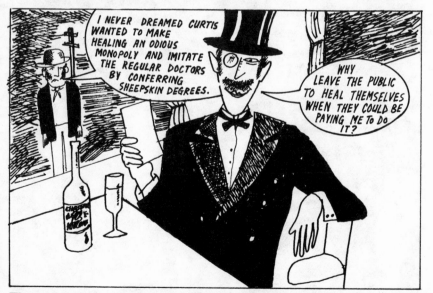

The techniques generated by the Popular Health Movement gained middle class respectability. Released from annoying democratic aims they quickly got monopolized by elites, and the movement petered out.

20th CENTURY DOCS

At the beginning of the century regulars faced competition from all sides. Apart from the numerous alternative healers, there was an excess of regulars themselves. They were being churned out by the many proprietory schools, the only entry requirement often being ability to pay.

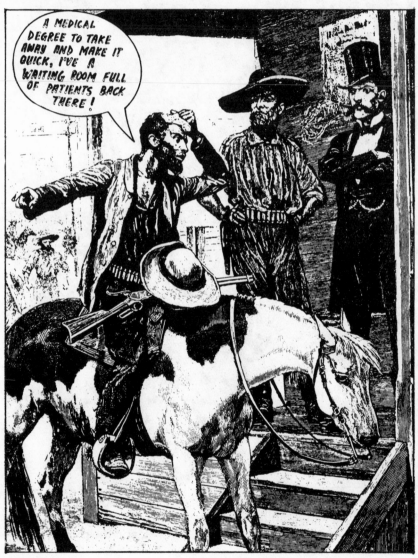

Diagnosis

> **The growth of the profession must be stemmed if individual members are to find the practice of medicine a lucrative profession.**
>
> Journal of the American Medical Association, 1901

But the American Medical Association had no legitimate reason to have its competitors proscribed.

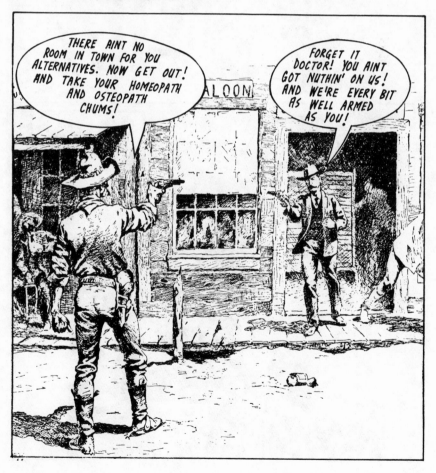

The AMA Felt Ill...

There was no effective cure in its repertoire. The prognosis looked bad. The condition clearly needed specialist intervention.

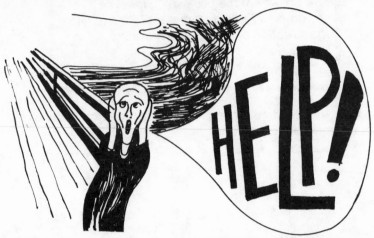

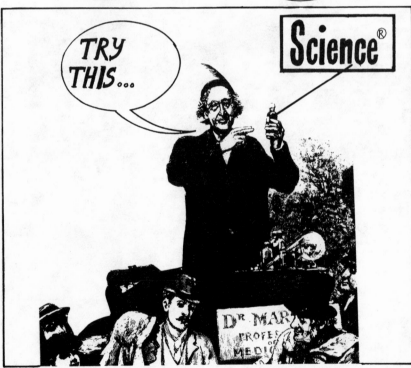

The Ideological Solution

The public was replacing religion with science as the legitimate source of truth.

The vestments of science would give the American Medical Association a special status.

In 1893, Johns Hopkins University put labs in its medical school, and staffed them with men committed to scientific research.

Labs were expensive. If they were made a requirement for medical schools, most would go bust, neatly reducing the number of doctors produced.

Salvation thru Science

PLIED SCIENCE

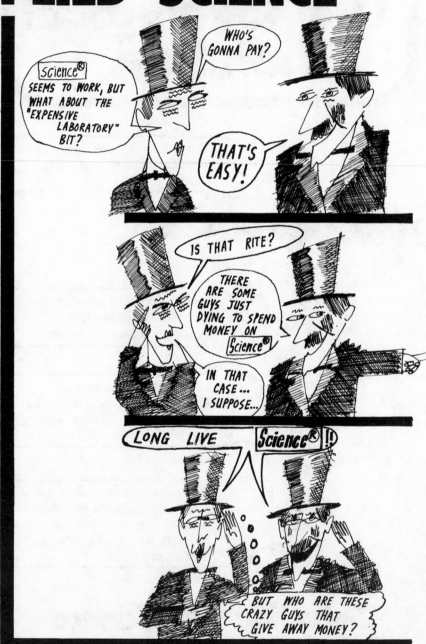

The guys who gave away money were the corporate capitalists.
Having accumulated colossal fortunes they set up philanthropies
to distribute their surplus cash.

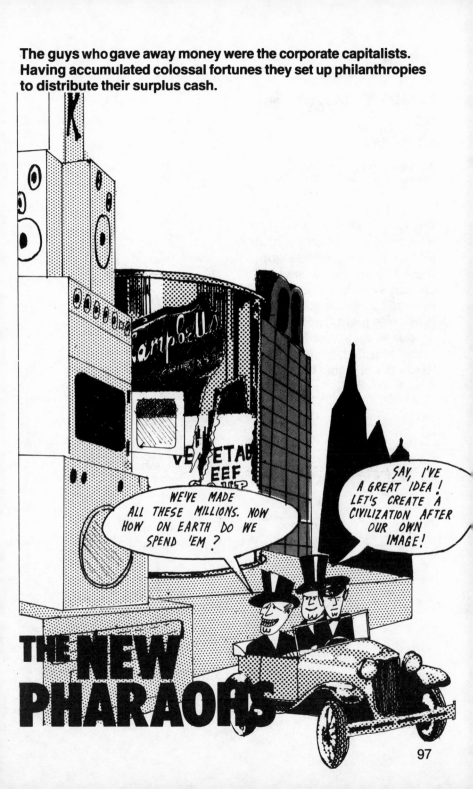

SCIENCE - what was in it for capitalists?

The new capitalists brought a new industrial ideology. It fitted into their mechanistic world-view. The engineers they employed rationalized the production process by dividing tasks into mental and manual labour along scientific lines. They thought a similar approach to medicine would be just as effective.

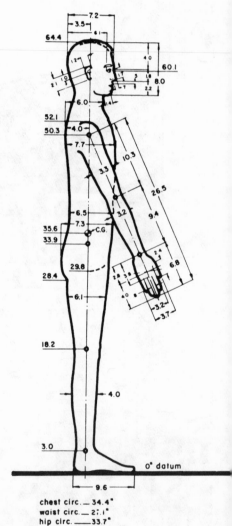

2.5 %.tile

chest circ.___ 34.4"
waist circ.__ 27.1"
hip circ.____ 33.7"

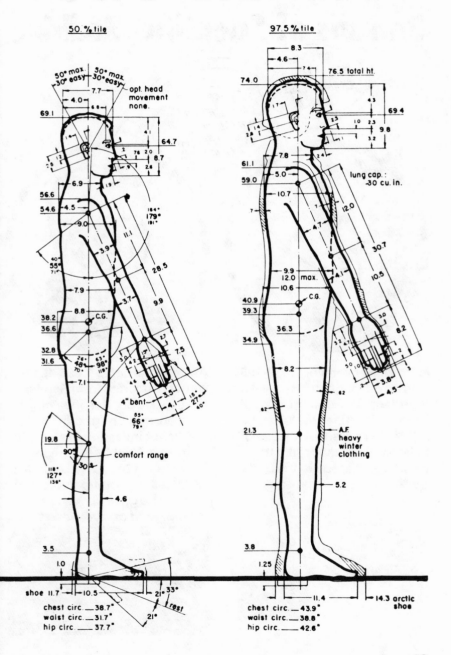

50. %tile

97.5 %tile

shoe 11.7 — 10.5 — 21° 33° rest 21°

chest circ. ___ 38.7"
waist circ. ___ 31.7"
hip circ. ___ 37.7"

chest circ. ___ 43.9"
waist circ. ___ 38.8"
hip circ. ___ 42.6"

THE BIG TWO
Patrons of Scientific Medicine

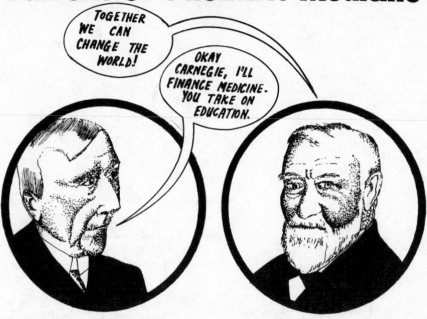

John D. Rockefeller (1839-1937) was an oil magnate. By 1880 his Standard Oil Trust ran most of America's refineries. When he retired his personal fortune of a billion dollars made him the wealthiest person in the United States.

Andrew Carnegie (1835-1919) went to America from Scotland in 1848. He got rich investing in oil, iron, and bridges. In 1873 he got richer investing in steel. The Carnegie Steel Corporation became the biggest in America. Ruthless with competitors and unions, he gave up his fortune for *the good of my fellow man*.

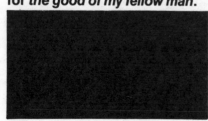

In 1892 John D. Rockefeller appointed Frederick T. Gates to administer his philanthropies.

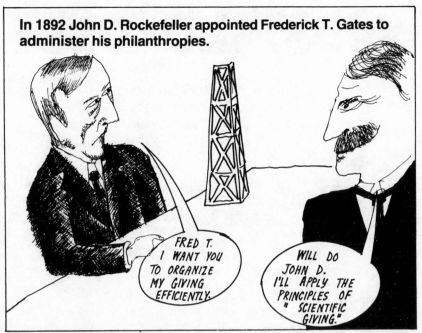

Gates was impressed by the fact that Pasteur's research had saved more money for France than the entire cost of the Franco-Prussian War. Though an ex-Baptist minister, he believed that <u>science</u> would remove all misery from the world.

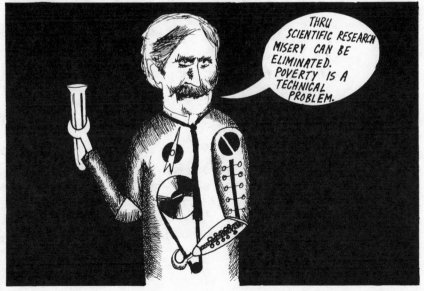

INDUSTRIAL BODY

Gates dished out large amounts
of Rockefeller money. His grants
were directed by his vision.

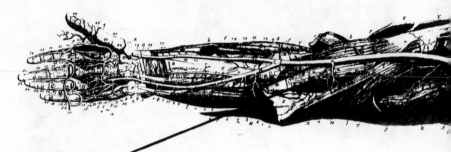

*The body has a network of nerves
like telephone wires, which
transmit instantaneous alarms to
every point of danger.*

*The great organs of the body are
great local manufacturing
centres.*

*The body has a most elaborate
sewer system.*

*The body is furnished with a
most elaborate police system,
with hundreds of police stations
to which criminal elements are
carried and jailed.*

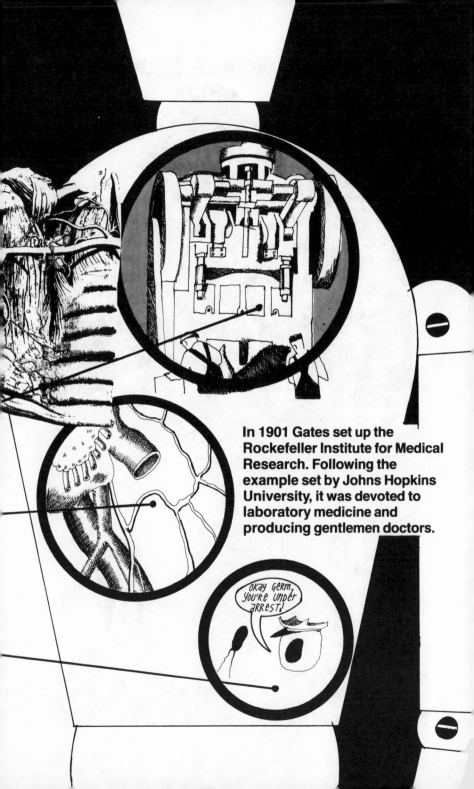

In 1901 Gates set up the Rockefeller Institute for Medical Research. Following the example set by Johns Hopkins University, it was devoted to laboratory medicine and producing gentlemen doctors.

The AMA wants more...

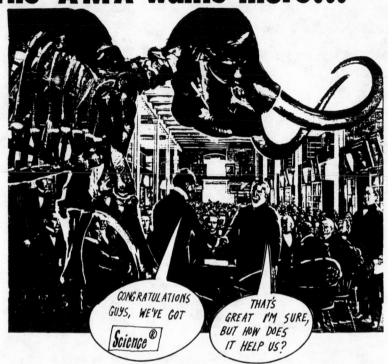

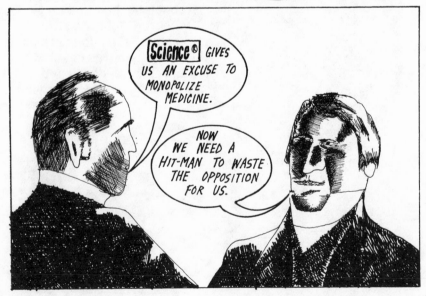

In 1907 the American Medical Association asked the Carnegie Foundation to survey all medical schools. Carnegie commissioned Abraham Flexner, brother of Simon Flexner, head of the Rockefeller Institute for Medical Research.

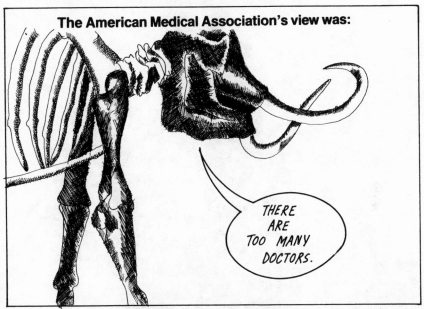

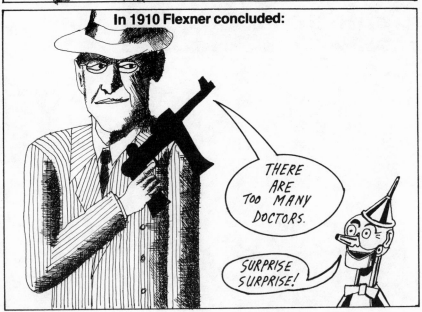

the
FLEXNER REPORT

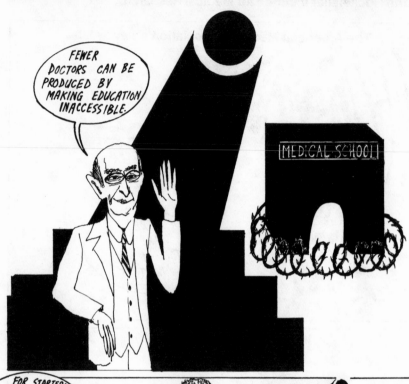

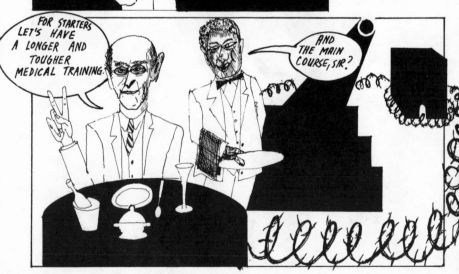

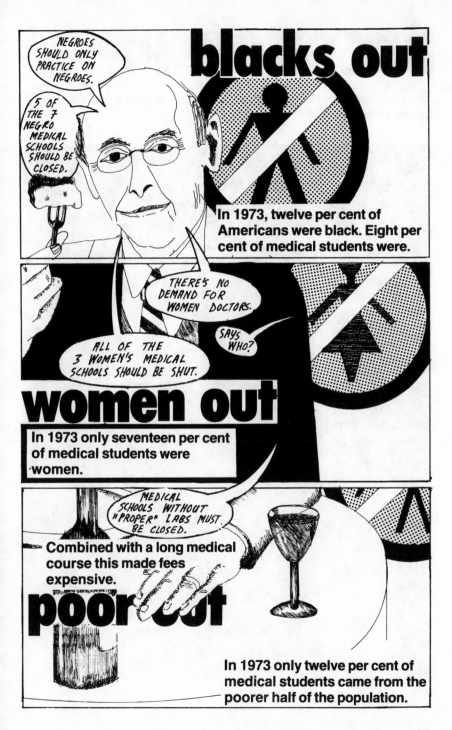

blacks out

NEGROES SHOULD ONLY PRACTICE ON NEGROES.

5 OF THE 7 NEGRO MEDICAL SCHOOLS SHOULD BE CLOSED.

In 1973, twelve per cent of Americans were black. Eight per cent of medical students were.

THERE'S NO DEMAND FOR WOMEN DOCTORS.

SAYS WHO?

ALL OF THE 3 WOMEN'S MEDICAL SCHOOLS SHOULD BE SHUT.

women out

In 1973 only seventeen per cent of medical students were women.

MEDICAL SCHOOLS WITHOUT "PROPER" LABS MUST BE CLOSED.

Combined with a long medical course this made fees expensive.

poor out

In 1973 only twelve per cent of medical students came from the poorer half of the population.

DOCTATORSHIP

The Flexner Report put medical power in the hands of a small clique of white, middle class, men.

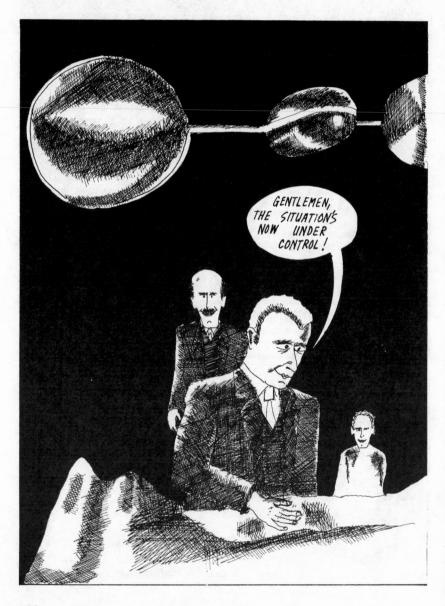

Dead-end?

By emphasizing laboratory medicine, it turned health-care into an expensive commodity. An expansive commodity that had a dynamic of its own. The voracious appetite of the process required ever more research and investment. Between 1962 and 1975 the proportion of the United States gross national product going on health-care rose from 4.5% to 8.4%. In 1975 $95,000,000,000,000 was spent. In spite of this boom in the health sector, male life expectancy recently began to fall.

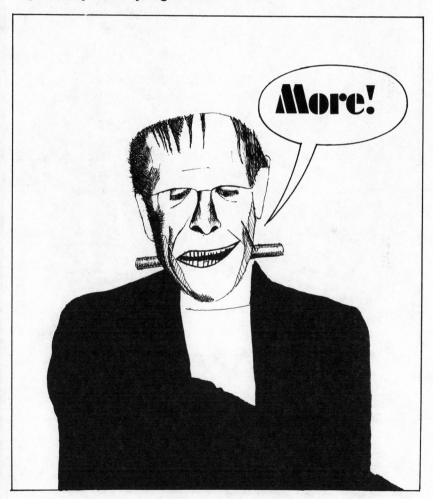

THREE

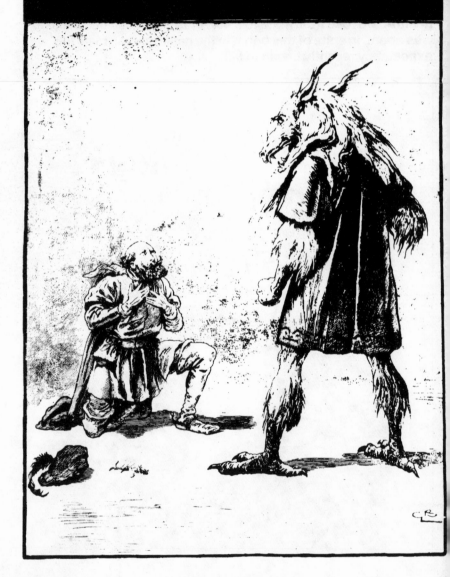

MEDICINE: THE UNSOCIAL FACE

19th century England

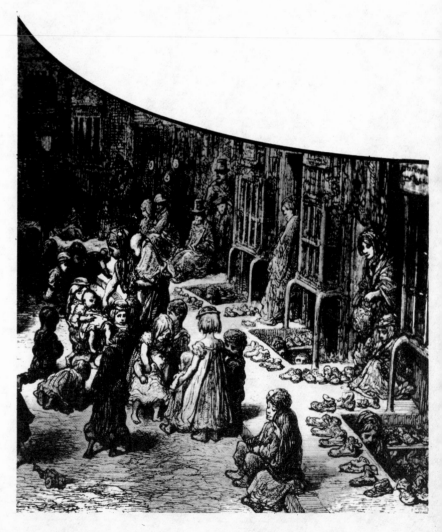

Before the twentieth century, five infectious diseases accounted for most deaths: typhus, scarlet fever, cholera, tuberculosis, and smallpox. When they declined, mortality fell. The medical profession didn't make the main contribution to improving health. Apart from smallpox vaccine, doctors had no effective way to deal with these diseases before 1935. According to Thomas McKeown, Professor of Social Medicine at the University of Birmingham:

> *The advance in health began in the eighteenth century and intially appears to have been due to an improvement in the standard of living. About a hundred years later this influence was supported by hygienic measures.*

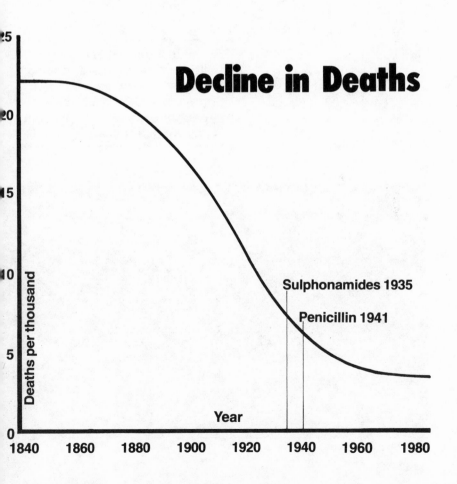

Decline in Deaths

Sulphonamides 1935

Penicillin 1941

Deaths per thousand

Year

1840   1860   1880   1900   1920   1940   1960   1980

25   20   15   10   5   0

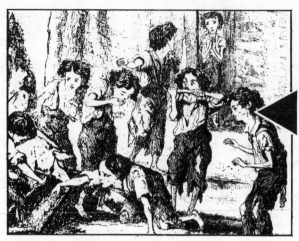

◀1840

1870▶

The main factors that improved health were better diet and living conditions. They resulted from higher wages. By 1900 real wages were eighty-nine per cent higher than in 1850.

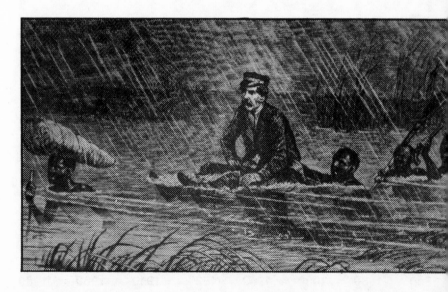

Worker demands . . .

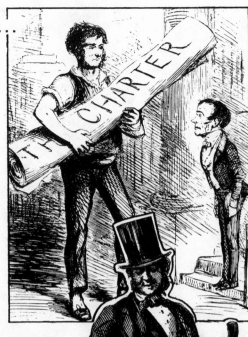

More productive equipment encouraged employers to pay higher wagers . . .

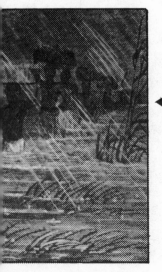

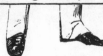

Colonialism brought cheap food and raw materials. British workers got some benefit and the colonized got the pressure.

1941... and beyond...

In 1935, the development of the sulphonamide drugs gave doctors the first effective weapon against bacterial infection. Penicillin was added to the arsenal in 1941. After the Second World War drug therapy came into its own. The atmosphere of hope that pervaded the post-war West included a belief that health would continue to improve as science advanced.

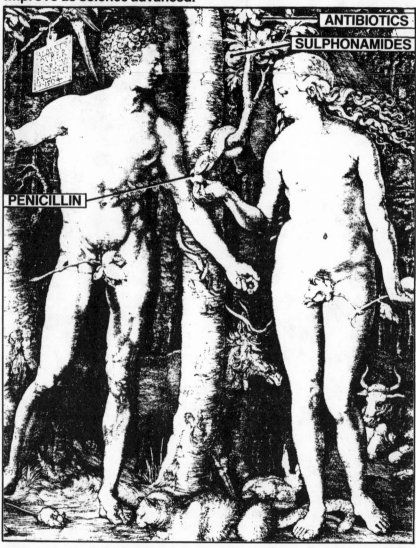

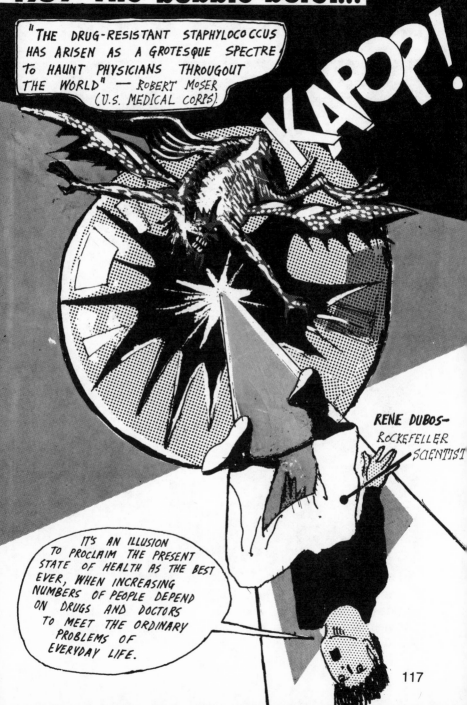

1962: Healing is dead; long live medical science!

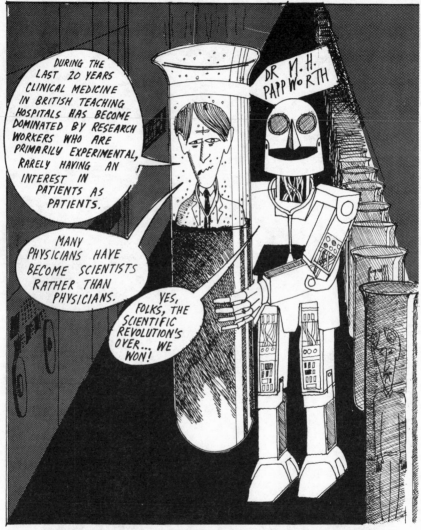

The prevalence of iatrogenesis – illness caused by the medical profession itself – became obvious in 1962, when deformed children were born after pregnant women had used the drug thalidomide.

1976: Ivan Illich

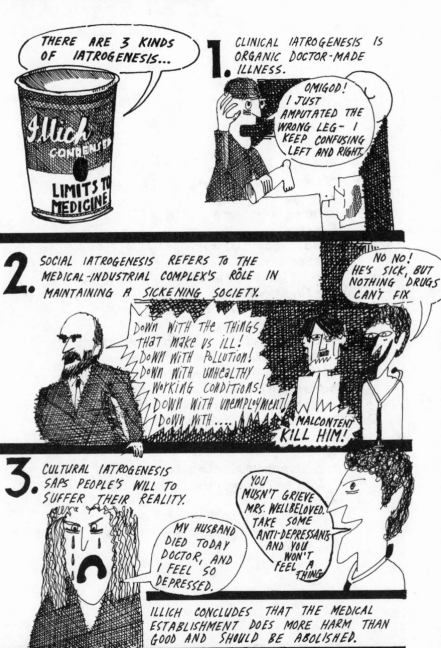

"Who are you?"

"I am Oz, the Great and Terrible" said the little man.

"I thought Oz was a great Head," said Dorothy.

"And I thought Oz was a lovely Lady," said the Scarecrow.

"And I thought Oz was a terrible Beast," said the Tin Woodman.

"And I thought Oz was a Ball of Fire," exclaimed the Lion.

"No; you're all wrong," said the little man, meekly, "I have been making believe."

"Making believe!" cried Dorothy. "Are you not a great Wizard?"

"Hush my dear," he said, "don't speak so loud, or you will be overheard and I should be ruined. I'm supposed to be a great Wizard."

"And aren't you?" she asked.

"Not a bit of it, my dear, I'm just a common man."

"You're more than that," said the Scarecrow, in a grieved tone; "You're a humbug."

Frank Baum: 'The Wonderful Wizard of Oz'

HEALTH & PROFIT

Health has become an extremely profitable commodity throughout the world. Although the British health service is nationalized, it still buys supplies from the private sector.

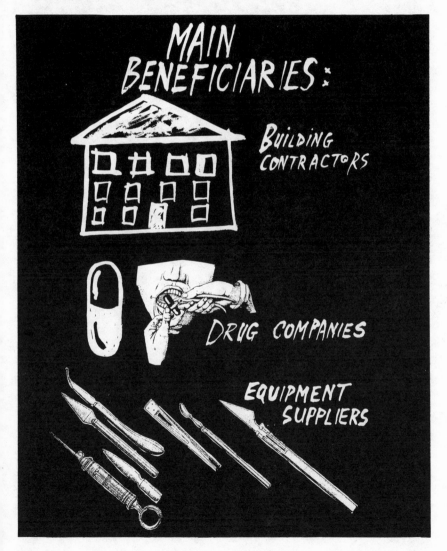

MAIN BENEFICIARIES:

BUILDING CONTRACTORS

DRUG COMPANIES

EQUIPMENT SUPPLIERS

Health or Wealth?

In 1977 the National Health Service in Britain spent £596 million on drugs.

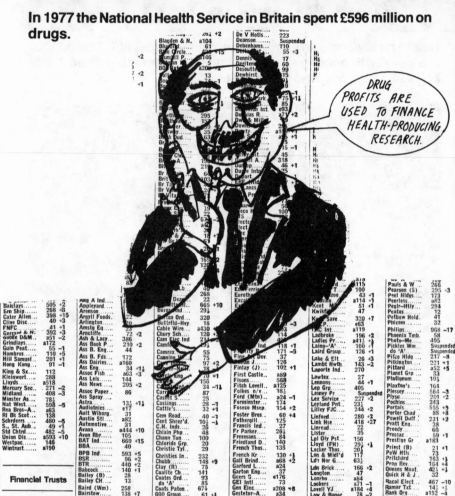

It is doubtful whether drug research contributes much to better health. In 1973, Henry Simmons, Director of the United States Food and Drugs Administration, observed:

> *The drugs age began to decline in 1956. There have been hardly any effective new drugs since then.*

Researching Questions

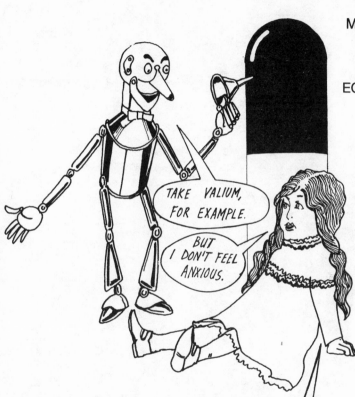

ANXON
TRANCOPAL
TRANXENE
TACITIN
NOBRIUM
SERENID—D
SERENID—FORTE
FRISIUM
ATARAX
MILONORM
TENAVOID
MILTOWN
MEPRATE
EQUAGESIC
EQUANIL
ATIVAN
LIBRIUM
TROPIUM
TENSIUM
SOLIS
SEDAPAM
EVACALM
ATENSINE
VALIUM

Valium is the most widely prescribed drug in the world. In the United States 47 million prescriptions were given in a year. Fourteen per cent of Britons take it. In addition there are tens of drugs that do the same job of reducing anxiety.

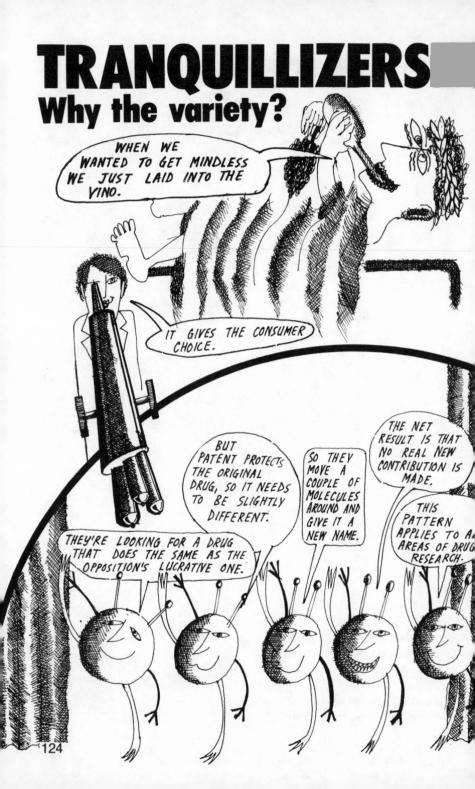

Why so much?

At the beginning of the 1980s, half of the National Health Service's spending went on psychiatric care.

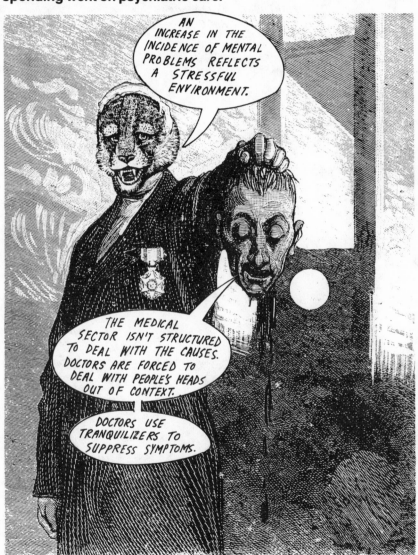

ANTIBIOTICS
Harmless wonders?

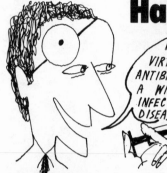

PENICILLIN IS A VIRTUALLY HARMLESS ANTIBIOTIC THAT CURES A WIDE RANGE OF INFECTIOUS DISEASES.

BUT SOME OTHERS ....

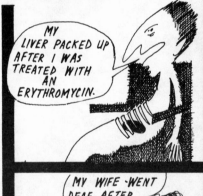

MY LIVER PACKED UP AFTER I WAS TREATED WITH AN ERYTHROMYCIN.

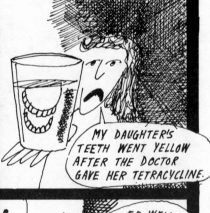

MY DAUGHTER'S TEETH WENT YELLOW AFTER THE DOCTOR GAVE HER TETRACYCLINE.

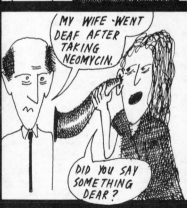

MY WIFE WENT DEAF AFTER TAKING NEOMYCIN.

DID YOU SAY SOMETHING DEAR?

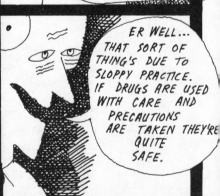

ER WELL... THAT SORT OF THING'S DUE TO SLOPPY PRACTICE. IF DRUGS ARE USED WITH CARE AND PRECAUTIONS ARE TAKEN THEY'RE QUITE SAFE.

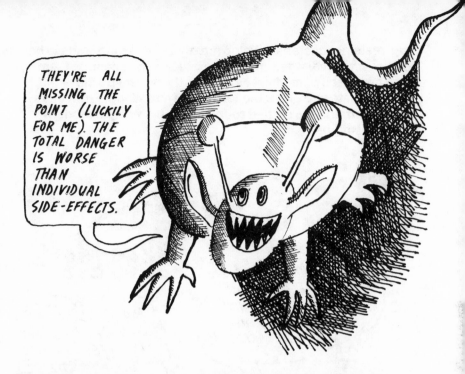

The indiscriminate use of antibiotics produces drug-resistant organisms. In 1981 . . .

Three quarters of staphylococci in cities were unaffected by penicillin.

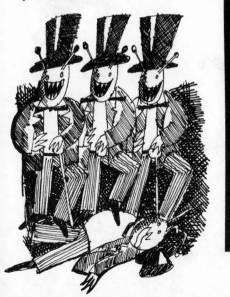

Half the cases of gonorrhoea were unaffected.

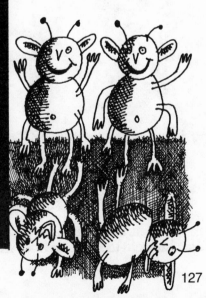

Drug-resistant bacteria develop rapidly, but there are limits to how fast new chemical weapons can be developed to combat them. There are cases of medical defeat, partly caused by the indiscriminate use of antibiotics in the Third World. From there, resistant strains are carried round the world by rapid modern communications.

THE Empire Strikes Back

In 1975 a strain of venereal disease that could destroy penicillin, was brought to England from West Africa.

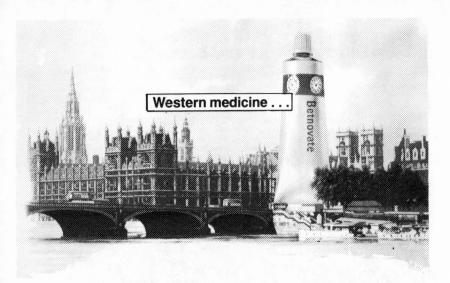

Western medicine . . .

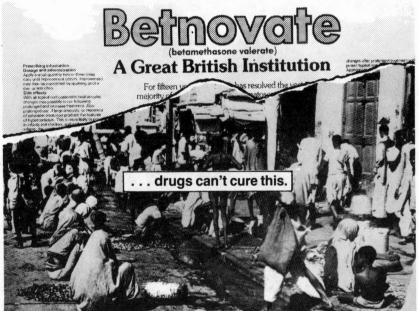

Betnovate
(betamethasone valerate)
A Great British Institution

. . . drugs can't cure this.

Current living conditions in the Third World resemble Britain at the turn of the nineteenth century. Sanitation, hygiene, and diet are inadequate. Curative medicine is inappropriate.

By the time Britain got drugs, health was already considerably raised through environmental improvements. Ironically those improvements were partly financed by the colonies, contributing to the present situation.

A COLONIAL HERITAGE

MALNUTRITION

NEW DISEASES

INSECT TRANSMITTED DISEASE

UNHEALTHY INDUSTRY

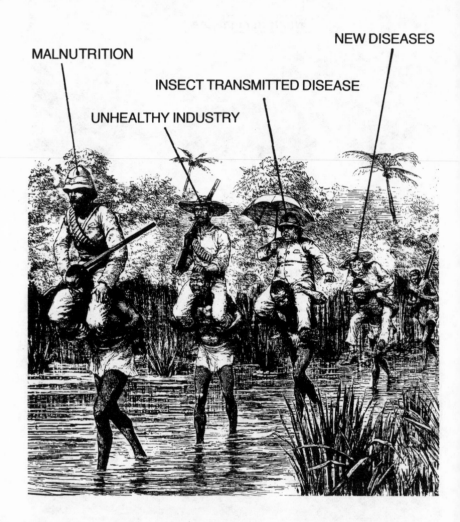

The major success of the World Health Organization disease eradication program has been the world-wide elimination of smallpox. However, before Western expansion, smallpox was unknown in much of the world. In the United States, for example, it was used as a potent weapon by sending Indians contaminated clothing or blankets. Not having previously encountered it, the Indians had no resistance to the disease.

It is widely assumed today that many Third World diseases have always been endemic. They are just thought of as tropical diseases.

AN EXAMPLE

In large areas of East Africa sleeping sickness has killed all cattle. Yet before colonization large numbers were farmed in these areas. African farmers controlled tsetse flies which carry the disease, a hazard to human health, by keeping their shrubland breeding-ground at bay. Routine bush clearing successfully kept the area safe. Through wars and then the imposition of the migrant-labour system, colonialism depleted the rural population. With insufficient labour to cut back the shrub, the flies moved in.

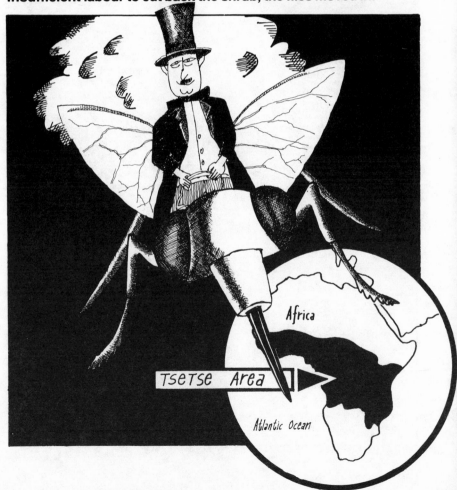

Africa

TseTse Area

Atlantic Ocean

GROWING FAMINE

Drought and crop failures undoubtedly occurred in pre-colonial times. After colonization, sporadic starvation through natural disaster was replaced by widespread man-made starvation. The cash-crop system is a major cause. Land previously used for subsistence farming is now cultivated for non-nutritional products, by multinationals. In fact, crops like tobacco, coffee, sugar cane, and opium are harmful, yet they replace the staples of the local people.

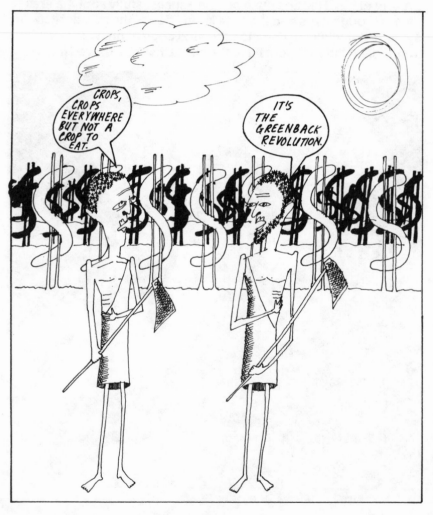

INDUSTRIAL REACTION

One attraction of colonialism to capitalists was the vulnerability of colonized people to exploitation. Once traditional subsistence economies were shattered, people became dependent on any livelihood offered. The creation of poverty forced the acceptance of low wages and often dangerous working conditions. Industries hindered by unions in the West could switch to the Third World where workers were less uppity.

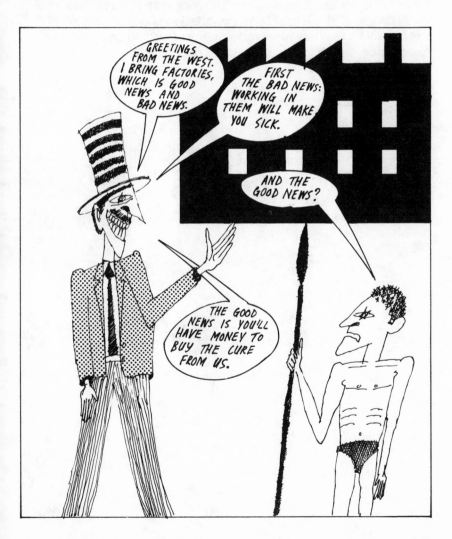

Medical Conquest
SUGAR-COATED PILLAGE

The West's style of curative medicine has been transplanted to the Third World. In the aftermath of imperialism, sophisticated high technology medical institutions have been set up. They continue the colonial relationship in a more subtle way, by making ex-colonies dependent on Western know-how and supplies to keep them running. The Rockefeller Foundation is one First World organization that has followed a policy of setting up centres of excellence, which impose industrial capitalist values on underdeveloped countries.

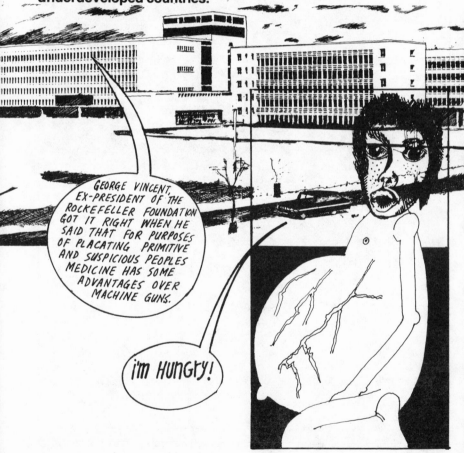

Profits of Doom

In the aftermath of colonialism, multinationals sell cures to the impoverished ex-colonies.
Drug companies dump drugs banned in the West as dangerous.
Equipment suppliers sell inappropriate technology to countries unable to afford it.
Buying from the West increases their debt and dependency.

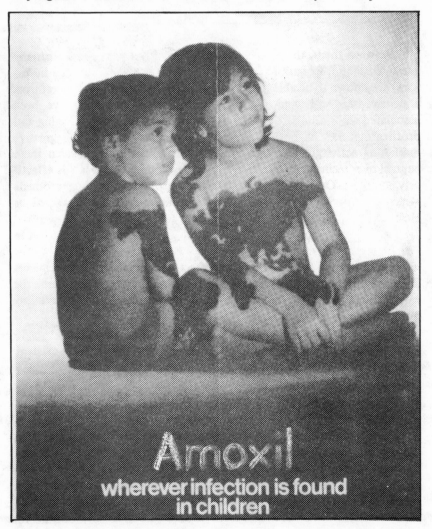

WHILE BACK IN THE WEST..
Food, profit, ill-health

Mass production of food has corresponded with falling nutritional standards. Less nourishing food is often more profitable.

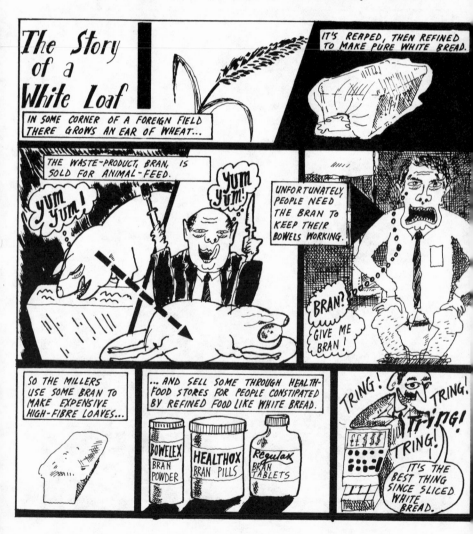

Social Drugs
ALCHOHOL TOBACCO
SOME PARTS THEY REACH:

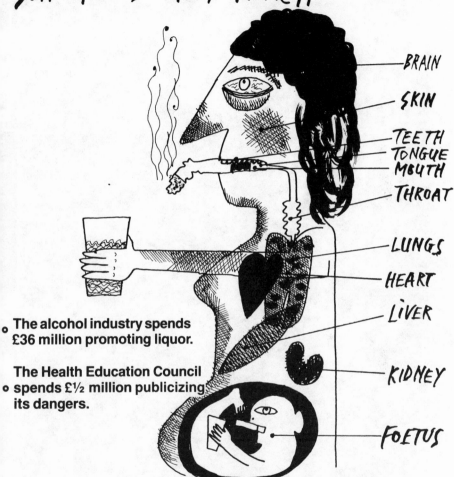

- BRAIN
- SKIN
- TEETH
- TONGUE
- MOUTH
- THROAT
- LUNGS
- HEART
- LIVER
- KIDNEY
- FOETUS

o **The alcohol industry spends £36 million promoting liquor.**

o **The Health Education Council spends £½ million publicizing its dangers.**

• **The Royal College of Physicians sees *cigarette smoking as important a cause of death as were the great epidemics*.**

• **A thousand people die each week due to smoking.**

• **Alcohol increases violence and accidents.**

• **In spite of stringent legislation in Britain, drunken driving is on the increase.**

137

Work Load

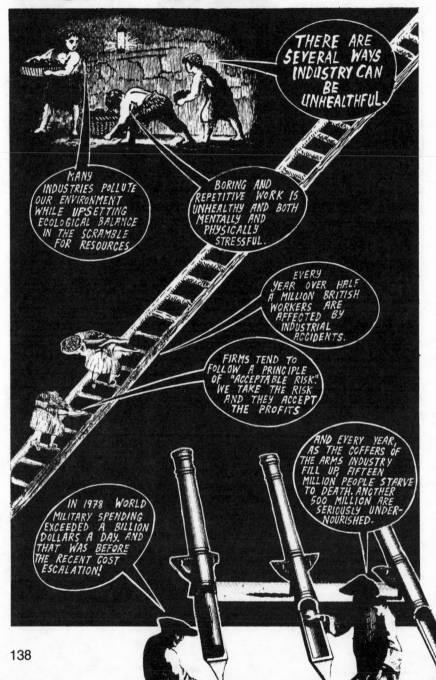

Dis-Ease

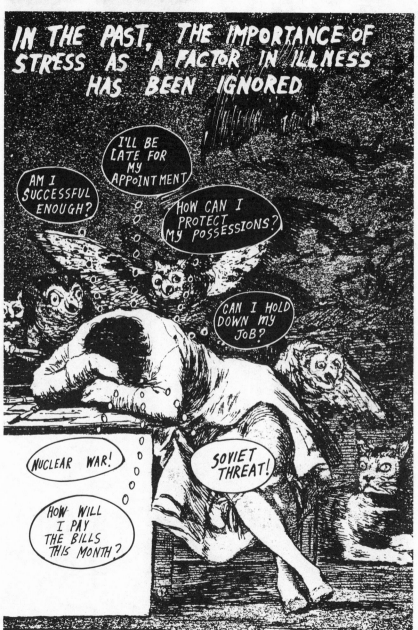

HEALTH & POWER

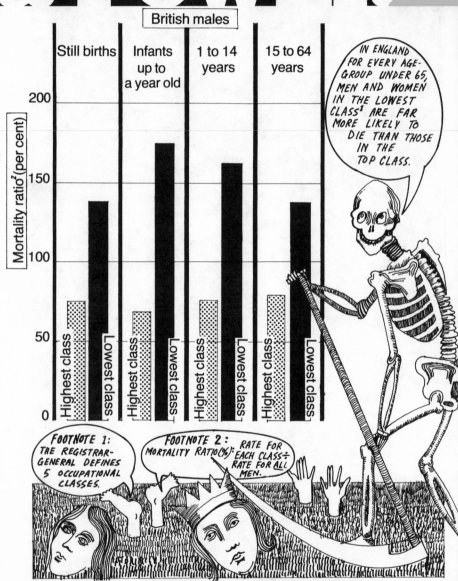

British males

IN ENGLAND FOR EVERY AGE-GROUP UNDER 65, MEN AND WOMEN IN THE LOWEST CLASS[1] ARE FAR MORE LIKELY TO DIE THAN THOSE IN THE TOP CLASS.

Mortality ratio[2] (per cent)

Still births — Highest class / Lowest class

Infants up to a year old — Highest class / Lowest class

1 to 14 years — Highest class / Lowest class

15 to 64 years — Highest class / Lowest class

FOOTNOTE 1: THE REGISTRAR-GENERAL DEFINES 5 OCCUPATIONAL CLASSES.

FOOTNOTE 2: MORTALITY RATIO(%): RATE FOR EACH CLASS ÷ RATE FOR ALL MEN.

DEATH THE LEVELLER?

MALNUTRITION

One big underlying cause of ill-health is malnutrition. It creates deficiency diseases like kwashiorkor, beri beri, and rickets. It lowers a person's general condition, and reduces resistance to all sickness.

Every year Americans spend $2,500 million on pet food. At the same time twenty-six million Americans are malnourished through poverty.

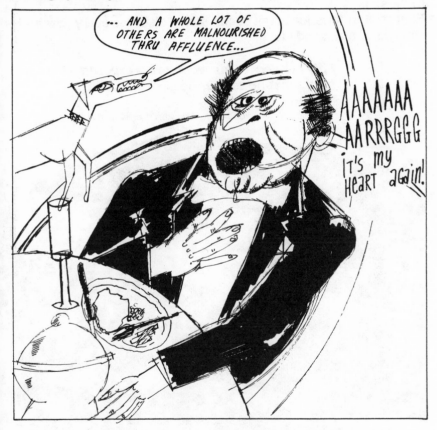

Hunger exists on a disgraceful scale in the United States.

White House Conference on Food, Nutrition, and Health

HEALTH UNDERMINED

- Coalmining is a major contributor to America's wealth, yet coalminers are the most illness-prone Americans.
- On an average, American mines kill a miner every other day. It's worse than the record of just about every European country – East or West.
- Four million Americans get occupational diseases every year and a hundred thousand die.

Fifty per cent of our workers are exposed to urgent and serious health hazards on the job.

U.S. Dept. of Health, Education and Welfare

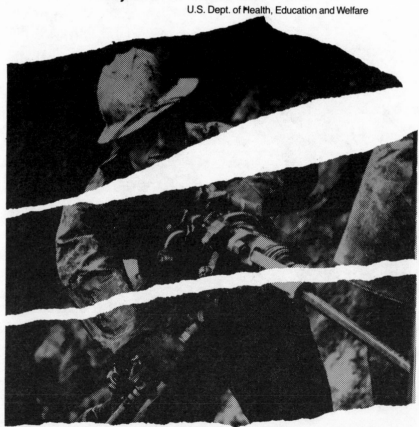

POWER VACUUM

The people in the resource-rich areas of the country are the poorest and least healthy. In 1967 corporations extracted from Appalachia $54 million more than they put in.

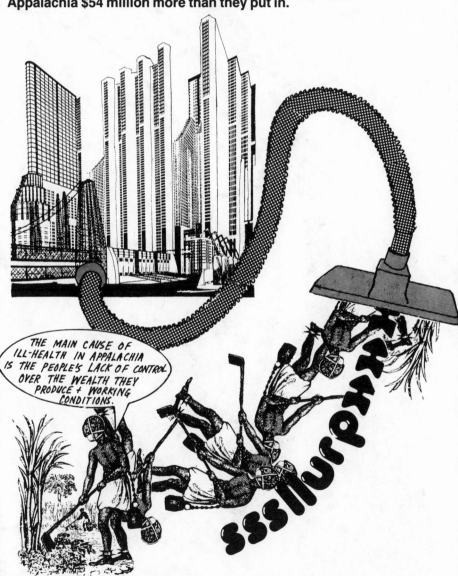

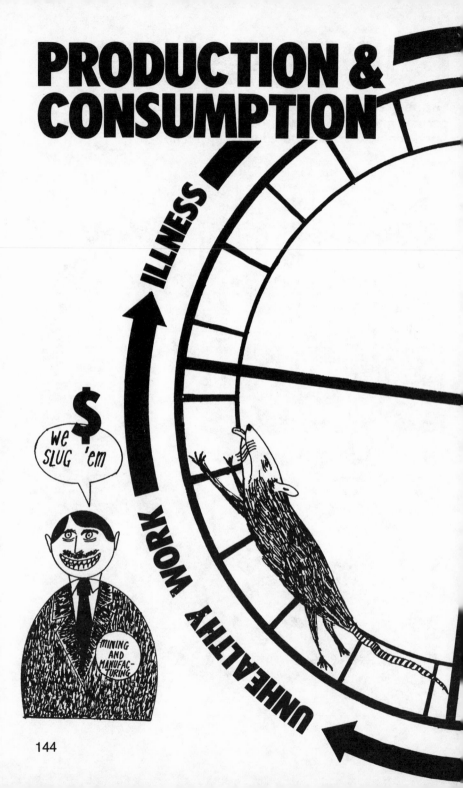

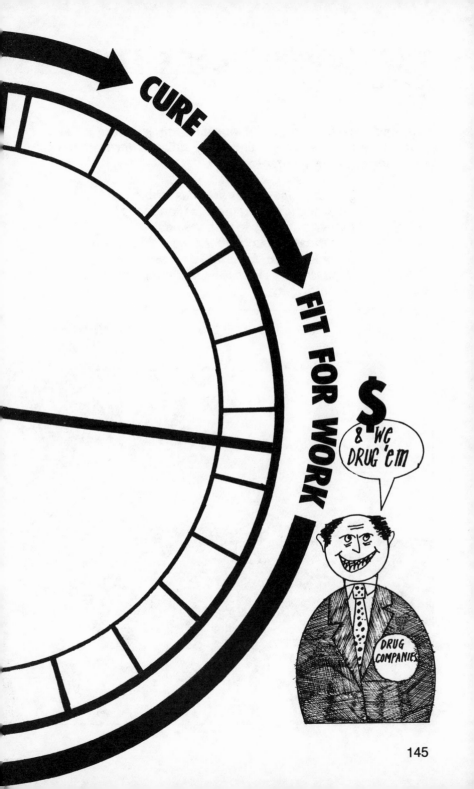

145

THE «INVERSE-CARE LAW» in the UK...

Despite the existence of the National Health Service in Britain, health care is unevenly distributed. Dr Julian Tudor-Hart explains this in terms of the 'inverse-care law':

> *Working class areas are a last choice for most doctors, and there is therefore a tendency for those with the best qualifications to go to the places that need them least and for unfilled vacancies to occur in areas with the greatest sickness and mortality.*

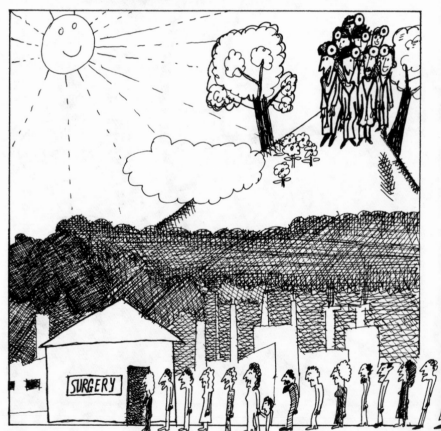

& in the US?

The same thing exists in the United States. Twenty-six per cent of its population lives in rural areas and is served by only twelve per cent of its doctors.

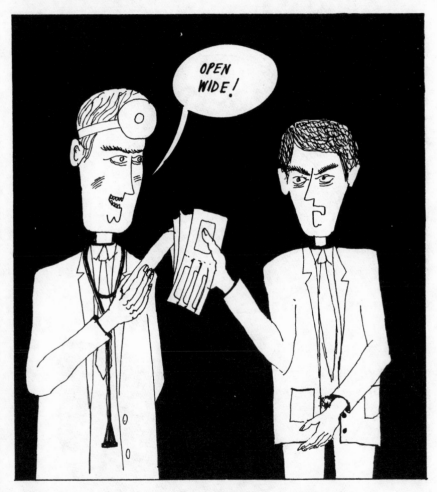

Fifty-two per cent of Virginian children had received no immunization against major diseases, according to a 1975 survey. In 1968, 60% of homes in West Virginia had waste disposal that was hazardous to health.

MINORITY RULE

The male domination of the medical profession reflects the male control of society at large. Although 70% of hospital workers in Britain are women, 80% of doctors, who direct the service, are men.

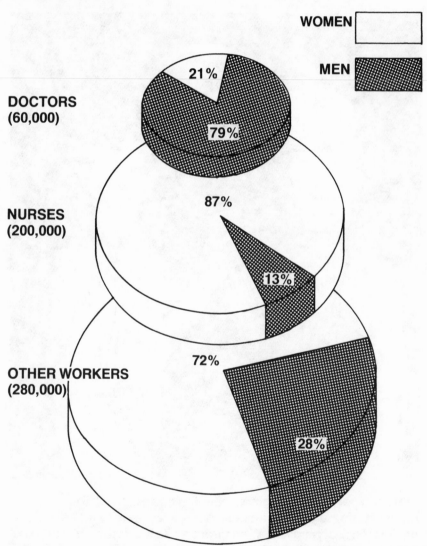

WOMEN

MEN

DOCTORS
(60,000)

21%

79%

NURSES
(200,000)

87%

13%

OTHER WORKERS
(280,000)

72%

28%

Masculation

In spite of a recent increase in the number of female doctors, the profession still holds an essentially male perspective. Women selected as medical students tend to show high ambition and academic achievement. As doctors they are encouraged to be objective, logical and resolute. The more "feminine" characteristics of caring, intuition and compliance are expected of nurses in the subordinate role.

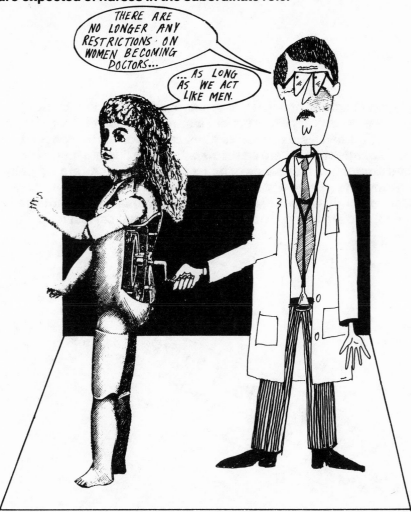

A FAST ONE

The prevailing attitude to women leads to complaints from some patients that doctors are patronizing and unsympathetic. This attitude is not new...

Medical theories of women have changed with society. In the nineteenth century when upper class men wanted their wives at home, women were defined as physically weak and in constant need of attention. There were few patients to doctors then. Now one doctor has thousands of patients. Consultations are typically around fifteen minutes. Doctors just don't have time for more. Conveniently, women are now defined as mentally and emotionally weak, and are treated with tranquillizers – medical fast food.

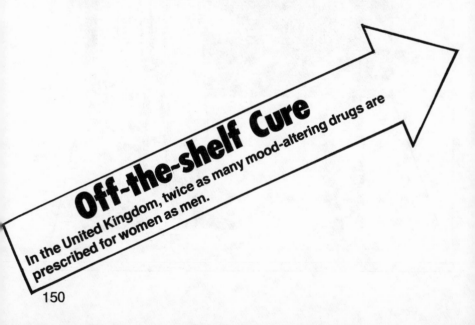

Off-the-shelf Cure

In the United Kingdom, twice as many mood-altering drugs are prescribed for women as men.

A woman's purpose is to preserve the family unit as a happy, secure place for both man and wife for the rearing of their children. Only by assuming this role can a woman throw off childhood inhibitions.

A 1971 Medical Text

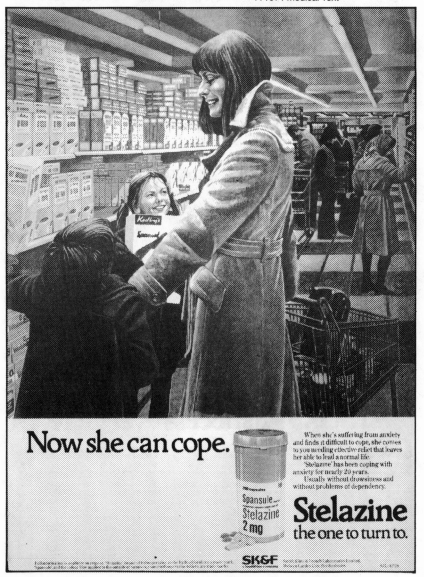

Wombs untimely ripped

Because of their biological difference from men, women are seen as medical problems. The word *hysteria* comes from the Greek *hystera* meaning a uterus. Hippocrates believed hysteria was caused by the womb's tendency to wander about a woman's body. He recommended marriage as the best remedy. In recent years obstetrics/gynaecology has become a highly specialized industry. Women's bodies are now the raw material for chemical and surgical interventions, often of unproven value. The surgical attitude leads to unneccesary fear of cancer in many women, creating more misery than it cures and diverting health resources into dubious screening processes.

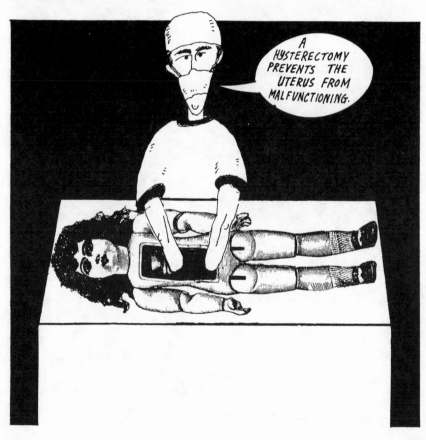

Smokescreen

Despite the fact that the Pap smear has doubtful utility towards diagnosing/preventing cervical cancer, the Pap industry flourishes. All this diagnosing breeds iatrogenic non-disease, wherein the physician treats his patient for a disease he has diagnosed but which does not exist.

Doctors Kothari and Mehta, 'Cancer'

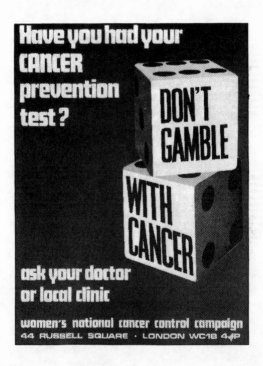

Screening tends to create a feeling in women that they are helplessly dependent on medical expertise and technology to stay healthy. Ironically many women demand screening as a right. They challenge the doctor's control of screening resources but fully accept medical assumptions about its effectiveness.

Bodyline

Even women's natural functions have become medical problems. Drugs are the answer for menstrual periods of all sorts: scanty, erratic, heavy, painful or depressing. And when they stop because of pregnancy, further medical intervention is regarded as essential. It begins with the obligatory rounds of ante-natal check-ups and culminates in hospitalization for the birth...just in case.

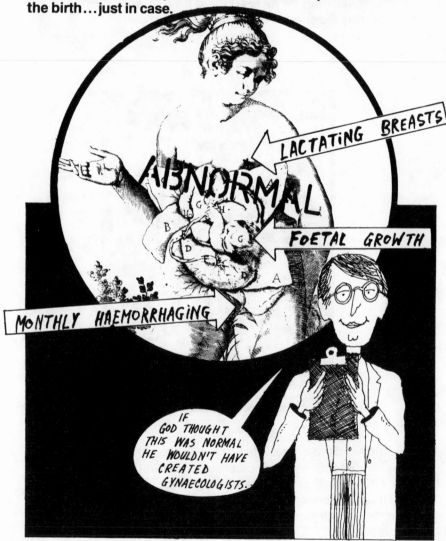

Ghost of Semmelweiss

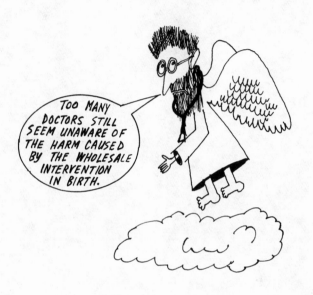

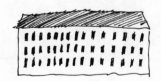

And the debate about the safety of hospital deliveries continues.

Maternal Triangle

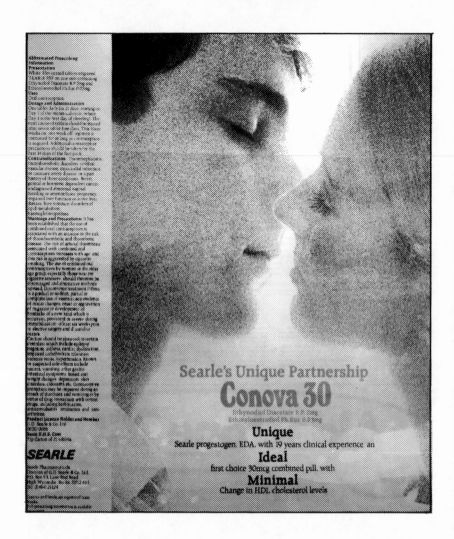

Searle's Unique Partnership
Conova 30
Ethynodiol Diacetate B.P. 2mg
Ethinyloestradiol Ph.Eur. 0.03mg

Unique
Searle progestogen, EDA, with 19 years clinical experience an
Ideal
first choice 30mcg combined pill, with
Minimal
Change in HDL cholesterol levels

**Modern contraceptives and safe abortions have liberated
women's sexuality from the consequence of pregnancy. But
this has not completely freed women. By law doctors decide
who can have an abortion, and by law they have the sole right
to prescribe many contraceptives.**

Healthy Response

Women are questioning the medical profession's right to withhold knowledge and to monopolize decisions about their bodies and lives. They are beginning to take control of their own health, and are taking childbirth back into their own hands...

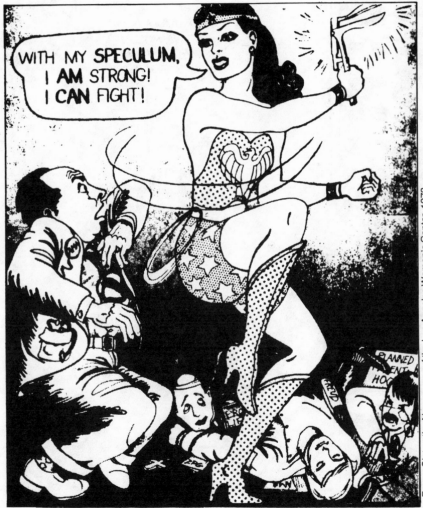

From: *Sister*, the Newspaper of the Los Angeles Women's Center, 1973.

Current medical science grew from a particular interpretation of the world. Since Descartes, dualists sought to dismantle the world in order to understand it. Having now reached the smallest particles and finding themselves unable to go any further, modern physicists are beginning to look to a new world-view that can take them further. This holistic philosophy is starting to filter through to medicine.

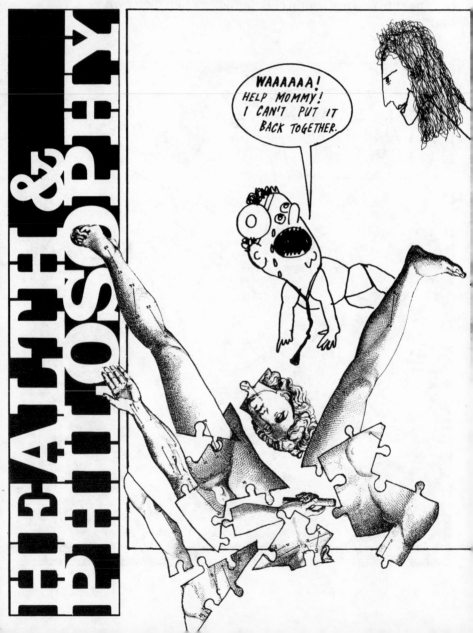

HEALING RELATIONSHIPS

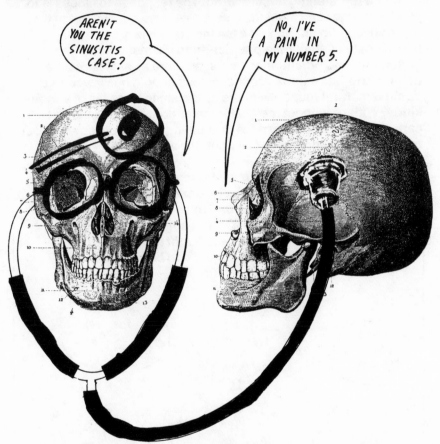

Dualism is an essentially mechanist philosophy. It describes a world of objects working as an elaborate machine. The approach has revealed much about diseases. But in so doing it has shifted the focus from the patient to the disease. Holists want to bring the doctor-patient relationship back into healing. In a world that has become a global village, holism seems well suited to describing the way things organically interconnect. It is not only pollution of the body that causes sickness, pollution of the outside environment is equally important.

The Message

The allopathic approach to illness reflects the feeling that we inhabit a threatening hostile world. The response to illness is to pull the trigger and blast the disease with chemicals. But in this war between doctor and disease the patient is often the unfortunate casualty. Malpractice suits against doctors are increasing and practitioners are seen more as assailants than helpers. Holists emphasize that illness should be viewed as a positive natural response of the organism to stresses of various kinds. With or without medical intervention, it is the inherent capacity of the body that does the healing. This process should be respected and encouraged, it contains a message:

> *To understand this message ill-health should be taken as an opportunity for introspection, so that the original problem and the reasons for choosing a particular escape route can be brought to a conscious level where the problem can be resolved.*
>
> Fritjof Capra, 'The Turning Point'

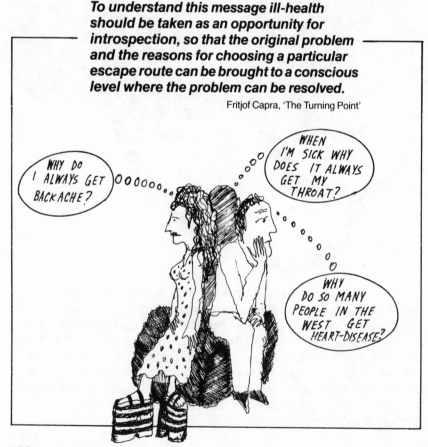

The Meaning

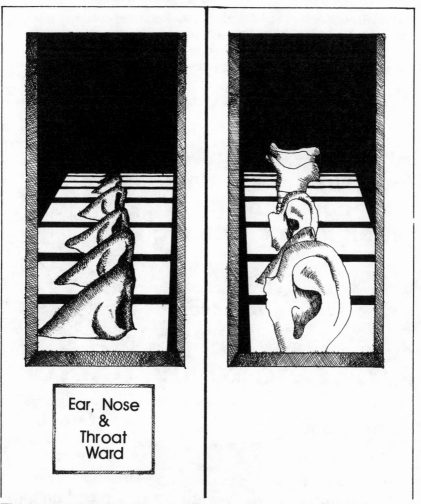

Ear, Nose
&
Throat
Ward

The increase of specialization has led us to lose sight of the context of illness in people and in society. A sick person is mainly concerned with his suffering and what it means to his life. Because of the rules scientists have set for themselves, they are unwilling to examine such things. The holistic approach takes feelings and relationships into account. By respecting each patient as a whole person in a unique set of relationships to the social and physical world, it tries to help them work creatively towards positive health.

161

epidemic proportions

Marcel Proust complained that for every disease cured by doctors they cause a dozen others, by injecting patients with the most virulent agent of all: *the idea that one is ill.*

Finns describe new disease

neurologists believe
discovered a previously

euphoric.
By April his legs were para-

in symptoms in early 1980
positive

Elderly who see lines bend should go straight to casualty

DON'T wait to get a letter of
referral from your GP – go
the casualty depart-

Professor Bird says, for
ple, that if the

ALLOPATHS CONCENTRATE ON PATHOLOGY. HOLISTS STRESS HEALTH.

Screening for ulcers

SCREENING for peptic ulcers by
ms of a questionnaire about
is prob

counse

Am I safe to fly, doctor?

Dr. James Le Fanu reports from the BMA symposi

ransport
symposium.
Even the well pressurised air-
a cabin altitude of 6,000

Warfarin resistance due to broccoli

AN unusual consequence of a cu

Communion brings relapse in coeliac disease

THE first communion of an eight-
year-old Italian boy caused a
relapse in his coeliac disease. The
presence of gluten in the communion wafe was probably responsi

Watch for sickle cell anaemia

GPS are being urged to be on the
alert for early diagnosis of sickle
cell anaemia.
Hugh Rossi, Minister for
that

for sickle cell anaemia th
facilities should be availa
either through referral by a
through special screenin
counselling cen

Cytomegalovirus cause of 300 cases of mental retardation

been confirmed that satisfactory for CMV infections in area affected

So what is HOLISM?

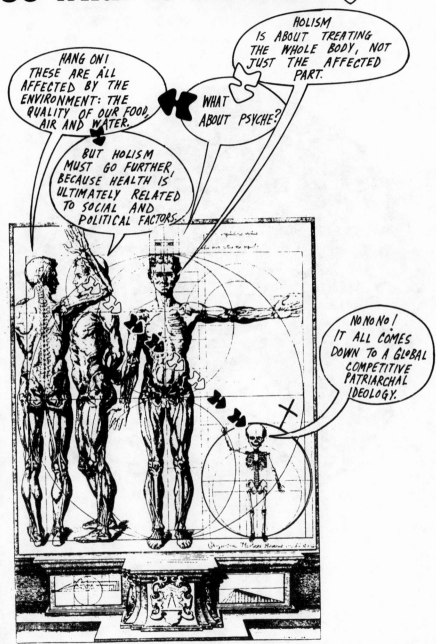

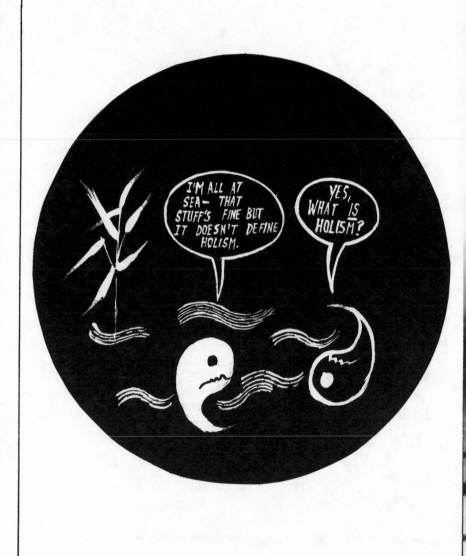

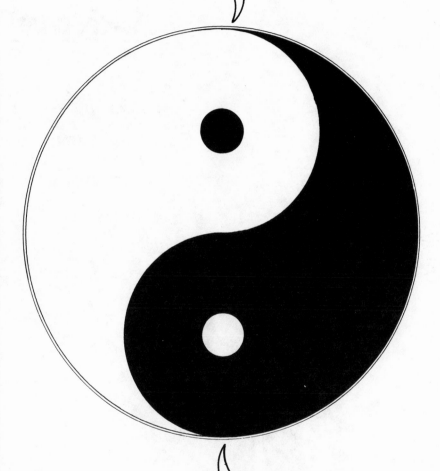

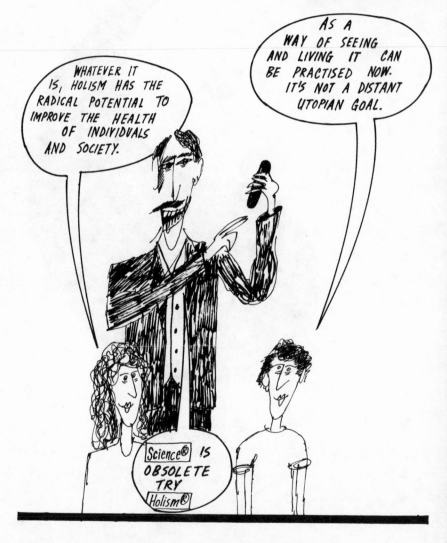

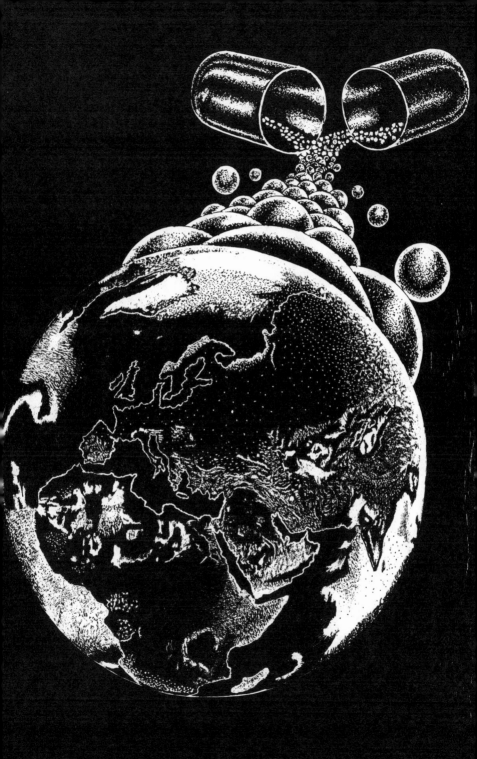

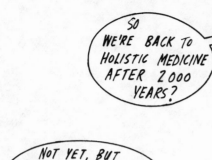

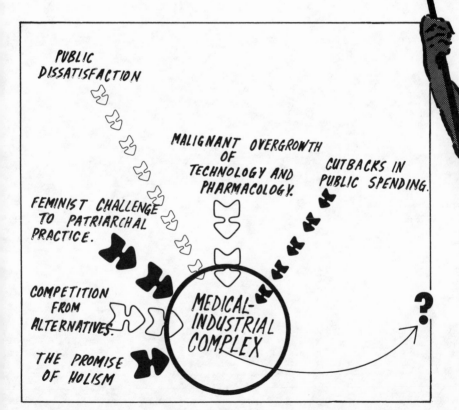

POST-MORTEM

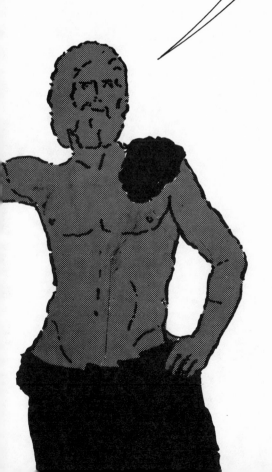

BIBLIOGRAPHY

Not a comprehensive list of works, but ones we found useful in making this book.

Miller, Jonathan **The Body in Question**. UK: Papermac, 1982. US: Random House, 1981.
A look at the way scientists have sought to understand the body over the centuries. His deification of western science can be taken with a pinch of salt. Good bibliography.

Inglis, Brian **Natural Medicine**. UK: Fontana, 1980.
A history of the rise and fall of drug-based medicine and the alternatives. Also a guide to the current confusing landscape of fringe healing and psychotherapies. Excellent bibliography and resources section, which lists organizations involved in "natural medicine" in Britain, Australia, Canada, New Zealand, and South Africa.

Inglis has produced a new book with Ruth West, **Alternative Health Guide** (Michael Joseph, UK, 1983), which is expensive but worth consulting because it brings his views up to date.

Ehrenreich, Barbara and Deirdre English **For Her Own Good**.
UK: Pluto, 1979. US: Anchor/Doubleday, 1979.
Full of interesting stuff if you can wade through the heavy style. About the rise of the medical profession through the suppression of women, and how the profession has defined and redefined women's illness to suit the times.

Navarro, Vicente **Class Struggle, the State and Medicine**.
UK: Martin Robertson, 1978. US: N. Watson, 1978.
An historical and contemporary analysis of British health care. Debunks the idea that the NHS is a result of the noblesse oblige attitude of the English upper class.

Dubos, René **The Mirage of Health**. US: Harper and Row, 1979.
A Rockefeller scientist exposes the myth that the key to health is to be found in the laboratory. First published in 1959, this pioneering critique is still relevant.

Illich, Ivan **Limits to Medicine**. UK: Pelican, 1977. Also published as **Medical Nemesis: The Expropriation of Health**. US: Bantam, 1977 and Pantheon, 1982.
This timely polemic provided inspiration and impetus for the growth of awareness about medicine's shortcomings. While open to criticism, it remains a challenge to disciples of the modern medical establishment.

Kothari, M.L. and L.A. Mehta **Cancer**. UK & US: Marion Boyars, 1979.
School of Illich. Two doctors attack the cancer research industry as iatrogenic. They call for a positive approach to cancer and try to provide alternatives to our disease oriented paranoia.

Weitz, Martin **Health Shock**. UK: Hamlyn Paperbacks, 1982. US: Prentice-Hall, 1982.
How to avoid dangerous and unneccessary medical treatments. Full of horrifying anecdotes. Enough to give any hypochondriac a real heart-attack.

Brown, E. Richard **Rockefeller Medicine Men: Medicine and Capitalism in America**. UK & US: Univ. of Calif. Press, 1980.
A fascinating study of the role of corporate capitalists in promoting the interests of the medical profession. Goes on to look at the current crisis in the American medical sector.

Doyal, Lesley and Imogen Pennel **The Political Economy of Health**. UK: Pluto, 1979. US: South End, 1981.
An excellent overview of the Marxist perspective. Covers the West, Third World, the NHS, women and related topics.

Ehrenreich, John (ed) **The Cultural Crisis of Modern Medicine**. UK & US: Monthly Review Press, 1978.
Readings on medicine as social control. Sections on women, and imperialism.

Townsend, Peter and Nick Davidson **Inequalities in Health**. UK: Pelican, 1982.
The Black Report, which looked at inequalities in British health, revamped. The government restricted distribution because of its unsavoury findings. It is now said to be the most significant piece of research into health of the last four decades.

Navarro, Vicente **Medicine under Capitalism**. UK: Croom Helm, 1976. US: N. Watson, 1977.
Essays on the destruction of health in the US and South America, and Marxist analyses of US health-care delivery. Also a Marxist critique of Illich himself.

Daly, Mary **Gyn/Ecology**. UK: Women's Press, 1979. US: Beacon Press, 1978.
The part about medicine relentlessly attacks the role of patriarchal gynaecologists in persecuting women. Bitter medicine for any man to swallow.

Capra, Fritjof **The Turning Point: Science, Society and the Rising Culture**. UK: Wildwood House, 1982. US: Simon and Shuster, 1982.
Describes a paradigm shift taking place in physics, and which is beginning to be felt in other fields including medicine. Interesting insights into the shortcomings of the scientific approach in medicine from a scientist, proposing new ways to think about well-being.

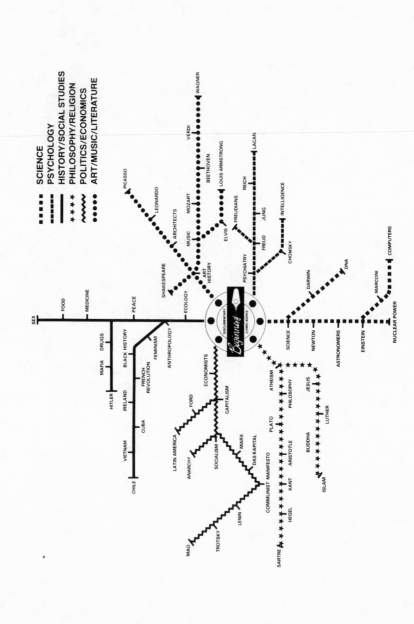